Sex Positions for Couples:

School of sex guide for couples. Tantric sex and sex positions for men and woman. Experience and training to get to know your partner.

By Paula Ann & Damian Old

Table of Contents

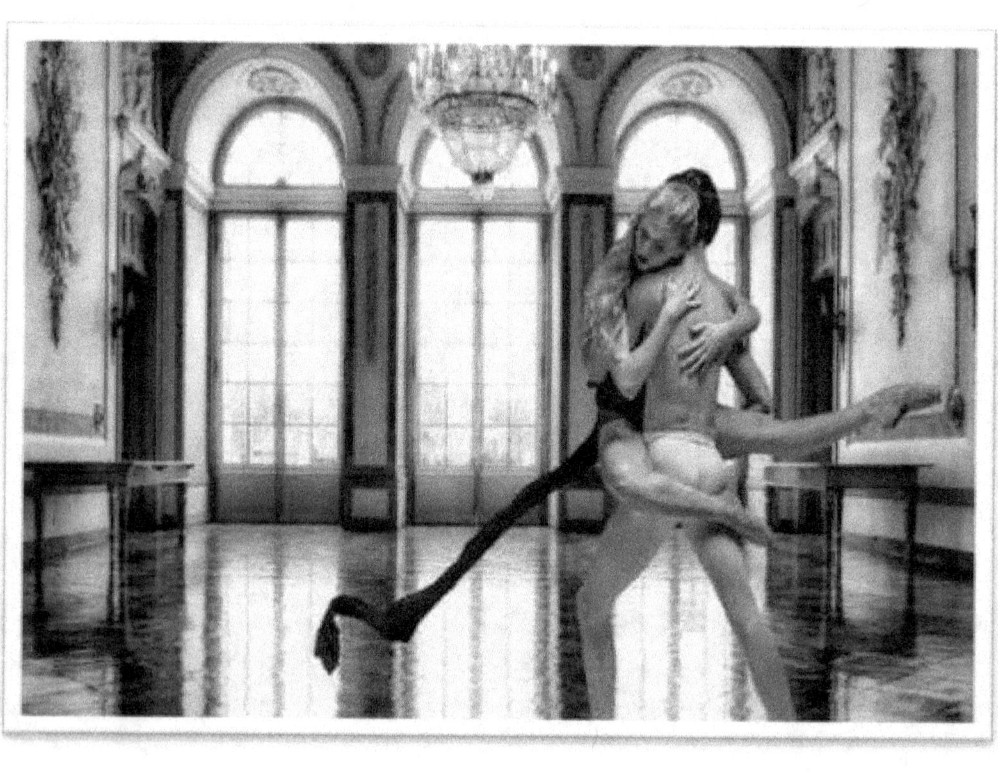

Introduction

Doing fun things together allows you to increase your dopamine levels together as well. When you have fun together, it increases your closeness with one another and can enhance the joy you experience with each other. It adds a unique sense of intimacy to your relationship that cannot be added by sexual experiences.

Ideally, you want to have fun together in a way that gets your blood pumping and your adrenaline rushing. Going to an amusement park, ice skating, visiting an upbeat concert, or otherwise doing something fun and exciting can increase the happiness of your experience with one another. Having fun this way can add energy to your relationship that will carry into the bedroom and make sex even more enjoyable.

Kiss More Often

Many couples, especially those who have been together a while tend to kiss less often. Kissing is a highly romantic and passionate act and should be done regularly. Think about it, at the beginning of the relationship you likely kissed your partner a lot more frequently than you do now that you are more comfortable together. You want to start doing it more often.

When you are kissing more regularly, don't just increase the volume but also increase the passion in each kiss. There is no need to peck and go. Give the kiss a few moments and truly experience your partner with each kiss. You can include your hands and body as well, or even kiss in other intimate areas such as on the cheek, forehead or hand.

When it comes to sex, the sex scene should be a fascinating and captivating one, though the longer people are in relationship a pattern is form especially when it comes to their self life. Partners sometimes find self doing one sex position over and over again. Well, one of the couple might find that regimen boring and want to step up to keep things new, spicy and refreshing in the bedroom, which is really how things with sex need to be with couples. It is fitting for couples to sometimes live and breathe experimental sex to bring forth a better connectivity with the partner. Behavioral scientist and relationship coach, Clarissa Silva opined that sex positions shouldn't be static for partners that need to connect for a long time in a relationship, but sex positions should always be learned, explored and practiced in the course of every connection. A lot of couples have put off their sexual flames just because of boring and monotonous sex positions which have made one of the partners looks else way to get the satisfaction and experimental sex he or she has always craved for.

Sex positions which are those positions of the body that people use for sexual intercourse or other sexual activities should be flexible, the fact remains that in an excellent sexual relationship a partner will want to learn and absorb all thing that pleases the other partner every time they both have sex, so that as the relationship evolves both partners will be in tandem, making it easier to be intuitive about one another sexual needs. The beauty of this is that you won't have to bargain what you need any longer because your partner will act on it. So sometimes you might not be lucky to have a partner that is experimental with sex positions but if not all hope is not lost. Aforementioned is why we have put together this book to help such couples out.

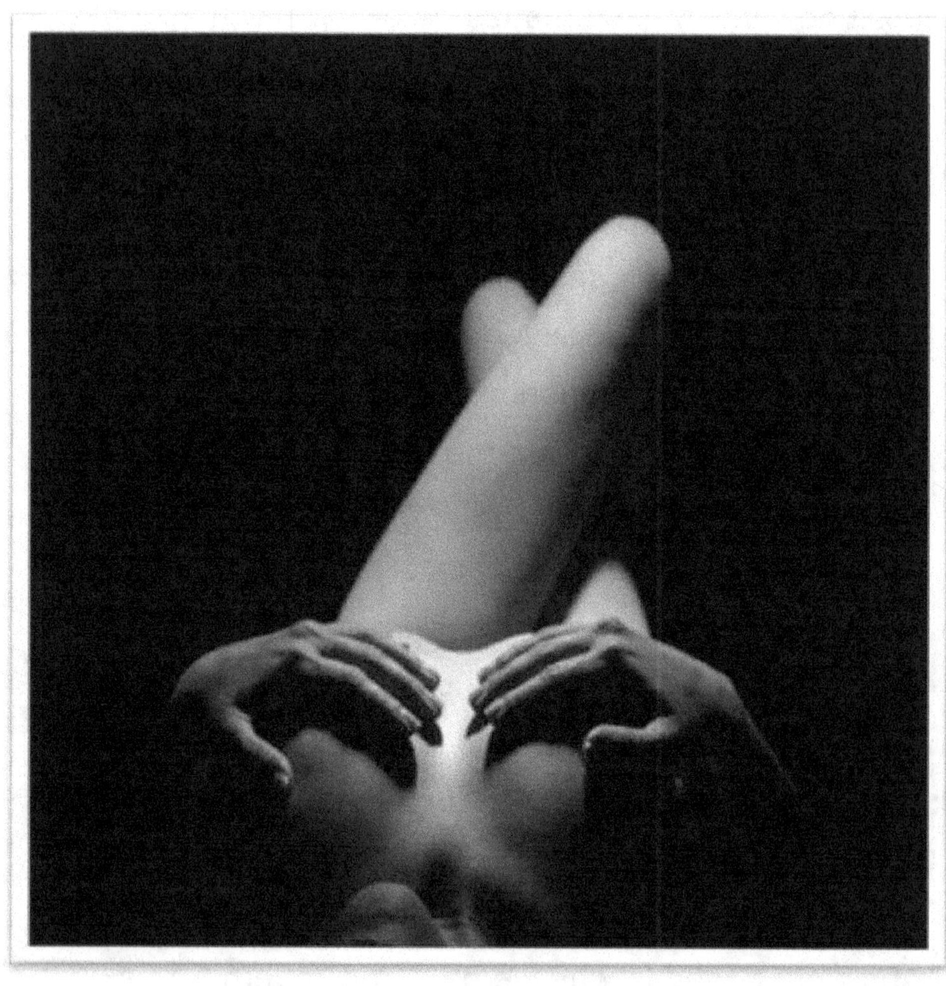

Chapter 1 Sexuality Today

Whether we are aware or not, it is common for people to vocally express pleasure and emotions during lovemaking. During sex, there are subtle sounds that convey various messages, such as wanting more. Every person vocalizes differently. Some people make a lot of sounds in bed, while others tend to be quiet and less vocal. The sounds we produce during sex affect our performance and our experience with our partner.

How We Communicate During Sex

Usually, TV shows and films depict vocals during sex in an intense way, and they often highlight climatic sounds of arousal. However, there are far more subtle sounds, movements, and gestures that can give much more depth to your sexual experience.

Non-verbal cues can indicate what your partner wants during sex, from engaging further to initiating a new position. Furthermore, the various sounds we make, such as a groan or grunt, can enhance our pleasure.

Let us take for example a bird that is about to take flight. It may chatter or vocalize its takeoff, do an embellished flapping of its wings, and extend its body. This behavior affects the bird's flying experience while also signaling to other birds that it is about to fly. This is similar to sex. When your lover makes grunts or groans during a lovemaking session, it means they are experiencing pleasure and letting you know about it! It might be subtle at first, and then it becomes more expressive. When you moan during lovemaking, it does not only give your partner an indication of your experience but also enhances your own sensation.

Vocals During Sex: What Do They Mean and What to Look For

How do we interpret the various sounds we make during sex? Some of the sounds we make are not initially made for the purpose of communicating but are more of a reaction to our own experience. The vocals we produce let our partners know what we want and how we feel during our interaction with them. The following are the different types of sounds and breathing that indicate various things.

Short, rapid breathing indicates a growing amount of excitement as arousal builds up during sex. Typically, this is the sound of pleasure as one partner begins to arouse their lover during sex. This usually occurs in the early stages, when initial foreplay begins or slips into a more intense exchange of touching, leading to sex.

Grunts and groans are usually sounds that occur during sex as a reaction to various techniques and movements, giving your partner an indication of how they are progressing. During lovemaking, we may not be able to explicitly say how we feel or direct our partners where to pleasure us, but when the reaction is a grunt or a groan, it essentially says, "Yes, right there, that's it." As the pleasure increases in intensity, progressing toward a climax, the moaning becomes louder, and we may clench our fists or contract our muscles.

Moans and other sounds that may indicate something completely different from pleasure (e.g., discomfort in a specific position) should cease. In some cases, a partner directly indicates displeasure by saying, "Stop, I don't like that," or, "I need to change my position." However, there are also times when they only produce a sound that can be interpreted as the same statement so as not to interrupt the general flow or progression of the lovemaking.

As your partner or lover reaches orgasm, the sex noise intensifies as well, becoming louder and sharper, often accompanied by the contraction of muscles. It is the height of the experience, and it signals that your partner has achieved climax.

Vocals During Sex: How and When to Use Them

There's a lot to consider about sex and the way you vocalize with your partner during intimacy. When you vocalize our pleasure, it can boost the confidence of your partner. They may equate louder moans and quick breaths as increased pleasure and being closer to climax, and this is why many women, close to 80 percent, admit to faking an orgasm in this way at least half of the time. This can cause confusion for couples who may not be keen on communicating openly about how they pleasure each other. It can mislead one to think they are adequately satisfying their partner when this is not accurate. On the other hand, when a partner is quiet and less expressive, it may prompt their lover to try harder and put more effort into lovemaking until they indicate their satisfaction.

How do we use vocals to communicate during sex to get the most out of pleasure and help our partner achieve their satisfaction as well? Be honest and responsive. Let your partner know when they are getting you closer to arousal. Vocals do not have to be overly loud or extreme. A few quick breaths and slight moans are enough to mean "Yes, that's it. Keep going." Or if a specific movement or action is not working, a simple "Let's try this instead" will do. You can also slightly adjust your body posture or position to change the method — that can work as well.

It is important to note that every couple communicates differently. While being more explicit to one's comments and description works well for some, other people are less inclined to explain how they wish to be aroused, or they are less likely to ask their partner how best to satisfy them. Having a discreet yet direct conversation with your partner or lover can resolve a lot of mystery in your sex life and make it a more open and enjoyable experience. If you are not sure of how to ask, wait until you and your partner are alone and in a quiet, comfortable space where you can approach the topic. You will be pleasantly surprised by how well-received an open and candid discussion about sex can be!

Interesting Facts and Myths on the Sounds of Sex

There is a big difference between sexual activities depicted by the media and those in real life. Oftentimes, in adult films or mainstream television, couples having sex are shown in positions that make them appear glamorous or ideal physically, even when they do not normally appear this way in real life. This extends to the sounds they make as well, where the louder and more vocal they become, the more aroused they are. This is especially grossly exaggerated in adult films, where the vocalization is overemphasized. What effect does this have on everyday couples? For people who regularly enjoy pornography, they may expect their partners to vocalize more than usual and achieve orgasm with little or no effort.

Some people think the louder the sounds, the better the orgasm. However, this is inaccurate in many situations. Some people are quiet during a climax. The success of orgasm is not measurable by the enthusiasm or crescendo of the sounds your partner makes. In fact, they may embellish things to give you the idea that they are reaching orgasm so that you will be satisfied in knowing you can bring them to that arousal. In reality, the loudest person can simply be expressing their pleasure despite being nowhere close to climax, and the quiet person may become less vocal as they reach orgasm. It purely depends on the individual, and it varies considerably from one person to another.

Talking dirty to your partner or teasing them with sexy whispers or comments is an exciting way to get them aroused. While this may seem stereotypical of film or sex scenes, talking dirty can definitely contribute in a positive way to sex and a couple's enjoyment of it. Imagine the reaction of your partner as you caress them with sexy words in the trace of a whisper. If you or your partner is new to this form of arousal, give it a try and gauge the response. Trying something at least once can be thrilling in itself and set the stage for more experimenting and fun later.

Communication is a complex process and involves the exchange of ideas, thoughts, and feelings. Just because someone talks do not mean that communication has actually occurred. If you have ever heard the saying "In one ear and out the other," then you know exactly what I mean by this. For communication to be effective, the messenger must impart information in a respectful, clear manner and the receiver must receive that message and understand it.

Communication is not only about what you say but how you say it. Body language and other non-verbal cues also play a part in the way communication works and how effective it is. Your mouth may say one thing but if your body language conveys a different message, then the communication process will be hindered. Sexual communication follows the same rules and is as equally important as any other instance of communication.

Being able to communicate your sexual needs and desires to your partner and vice versa facilitates a more rewarding and satisfying sex life. There is the largely mistaken assumption that if two people are in love and sexually attracted to each other, then the pieces will fall into place without being spoken about. That is not so, even if you two are sexually compatible. Just to determine sexual compatibility, open communication and dialogue are needed simply because no two people have completely harmonious sexual needs.

Communication can be abused. Some people are master manipulators in using the process to get what they want. When choosing a sexual partner and engaging in sexual communication, it is important to know that your partner is trustworthy and considerate of your needs. Do not engage in any sexual activity with someone whose intentions you are unsure of.

With that being said, let's move on to the types of sexual communication and how important each is. There are different stages of communication needed for a relationship to develop in a healthy manner. They include:

- **Communication during the early stages of a relationship**. Remember that open communication is needed in the earliest stages of relationship to determine sexual compatibility and whether or not this is a deal-breaker for either party. Flirting is often the strongest during the early parts of a relationship, and this, too, is a form of sexual communication. Flirting allows both parties to express their interest in the other and to determine whether or not their interest is reciprocated. Sexual communication in the early part of a relationship also opens the door for sexual negotiation for each party to determine how far each will proceed in certain types of sexual engagement or what activities each will engage in with the other.

- **Communication on health.** The incidence of contracting sexually transmitted diseases such as HIV and AIDS continues to rise every day, and thus, it is very important that you engage in open dialogue with your partner about safe sex and each other's sexual history for both their safety and yours. Some people find engaging in this discussion topic embarrassing and awkward and shy away from the discussion. However, it is a discussion that needs to be had for mutual wellbeing.

- **Sexual communication for established relationships.** This applies to persons who are seriously dating, engaged, and married and is needed to facilitate mutual satisfaction in the relationship's sexual affairs. When a couple reaches this stage in the relationship, it is likely that the couple has already engaged in sex. Therefore, communication at this stage is about fine-tuning the experience for both parties. It is about full disclosure of how your partner's sexuality and sexual actions affect you and vice versa.

How To Vocalize Your Sexual Needs

Communication about sexual needs is one of the most challenging parts of establishing a relationship despite the possibility that it has the potential to be an intimate and romantic process. It involves being comfortable and trusting your partner enough to disclose your needs and wants. By not doing so, you run the risk of having a very unsatisfying sex life and developing an unhealthy resentment toward your partner since your needs are not being met. However, you cannot blame your partner if you have not vocalized your sexual needs. Therefore, this section is dedicated to showing you how to vocalize your sexual needs in a way that is respectful yet commands attention.

Before you even get to discussing anything with your partner, you need to take a moment for introspection. You need to first know what your needs are and to accept them. You can read books or watch educational sexual programs to understand the physical, emotional, and mental sexual needs that you have. Even watching pornography can give you insight into your sexual needs and wants.

After you have more of an insight into what makes you tick sexually then you can broach the subject with your partner. Most people have grown up being uncomfortable and embarrassed about discussing sexual needs and, therefore, fear that they might be rejected or humiliated by revealing their desires. However, you need to get over that fear because your partner is not a mind-reader and needs to be told explicitly what you like and what you do not like. You need to let your partner know what you find comfortable doing, what pleases you most, what makes sexual encounters better for you, and what you do not enjoy at all. Do not rely on getting this information off the top of your head. Record it in some way so that you can have it handy for discussion when you do broach the subject with your partner

Before you start an open dialogue with your partner, you need to prepare both of you for that conversation so that you approach with a sense of curiosity rather than of defensiveness. Ensure that this is one-on-one time together with no interruptions and in a setting that encourages intimacy. Having a dinner date or going for a walk are great ways of introducing talks about your sexual needs. Planning a trip to a new location is an even better idea since you are already exploring new things. What would be better than exploring new parts of your sexual life together? Being in a new environment increases the possibility of having new meaningful encounters together compared to being in an environment that you are both familiar with. No matter where you choose to bring up the subject of your sexual needs with your partner, it is imperative that you place thought on the location as it can determine whether or not your partner reacts negatively or positively to the discussion.

There are good ways of broaching the subject and, of course, ways that do not encourage a positive response. Below you can find a few suggestions and guidelines to make vocalizing your sexual needs to your partner easier for both of you:

•	Start the discussion off by being prepared to talk openly and to listen to what your partner has to say.

•	Never compare your partner or relationship with a former lover or relationship.

•	Do not start sentences with "you do not…," "you never…," or "you always…" since this will only put off your partner

•	If your partner does react defensively, try to keep calm and not react negatively. Instead, encourage your partner to remain level-headed and open to the discussion.

•	Gentle ways of opening the discussion would be to say things like, "it gets me excited when…," "I would love it if you…," "I have a fantasy about…," and "I think it would be fun if…"

Just as it is important to vocalize your needs to your partner, it is important not to presume that you know exactly what your partner likes and wants from you sexually. Just as you have vocalized your needs and wants, create a safe space and environment for your partner to do the same. Encourage them to open up to you by asking questions such as:

- Are there any erotic scenes from movies that really turn you on?

- Is there anything that you did when you were younger but have not tried in a while but would be interested in revisiting?

- Is there anything you would like me to do for you sexually?

- Is there anything that you find particularly enjoyable or would like me to do more?

- Are you interested in acts of submission and domination such as getting tied up or blindfolded?

More Tips on How to Communicate Your Sexual Needs and Desires

- **Write down your desires.** If you find it difficult to vocalize your needs then try writing them down in the form of a letter and exchanging it with your partner.

- **Let your hands do the talking for you.** While engaged in sexual encounters with your partner, you can simply place their hand in the right place by guiding it with yours to show them what you like.

- **Give brief instructions during sexual encounters.** Use words like faster, slower, and harder to quickly and efficiently let your partner know what you need during the act. You can let your partner know when he or she gets it right by giving positive feedback and saying things such as "Yes, just like that" or "That feels very good."

- **Read and watch books and programs that aid your sex life.** There are many sex manuals out there that you can peruse together to find useful solutions and ideas to spice up your sex life. The same is true about sexual programs. After the two of you have educated yourself, then you can have a discussion on topics or ideas that were of particular interest to both of you.

Creating Sexual Intuition

In our everyday lives, we rely on intuition to guide us, especially in situations where we are unfamiliar or do not have experience. Intuition is defined as the ability to understand something or a situation instinctively without the need for conscious reasoning. Sometimes it is referred to as a hunch or a gut feeling. Everyone has some level of intuitive ability, and it can be thought of to be a sixth sense.

Intuition is something that is also present in our sex lives, and in sexual situations, it is referred to as sexual intuition. This particular intuition can manifest itself in the form of attraction to certain people or awareness of someone's feelings without spoken communication. It can also manifest itself in knowing just how to help and comfort your partner without them having to say anything. Having sexual intuition is a powerful thing as it can foster the development of deeper levels of intimacy and trust. With awakened sexual intuition, you can listen to your partner's nonverbal cues and respond in a way that allows you both to feel more connected with each other. Sexual intuition elevates the feelings that are aroused during lovemaking and makes orgasms more intense because of the increased sensitivity to each other's needs.

While some people have this intuition when it comes to engaging in sexual encounters, it does not come naturally to most people. The good news is that it is something that can be developed with time and experience.

As you develop your sexual intuition, you will be able to see signs and messages in your interactions with your partner that allow you to know that you are on the right track in your sexual relationship or activities. Such signs include your partner's body language. Does your partner lean into you when you touch them? Do goosebumps pop up on their skin when you kiss?

By being in tune with your partner's responses to the things that you do and don't do, you can develop the intuition or gut reaction to let you know how to give them the pleasure they need during sexual encounters. Just as there are positive nonverbal cues like blushing and an increased breathing rate, there are also negative ones that allow you to know that you should back off such as tense shoulders, a set in the lips or your partner refusing to make eye contact. Being more communicative with your lovers, past and present, allows you to observe patterns in their actions that allow you to understand the sexual needs and preferences. Educating yourself with books and sexual programs can also develop your sexual intuition as this allows you to look for certain signs when you engage in sex with your partner and to understand what these signs likely mean.

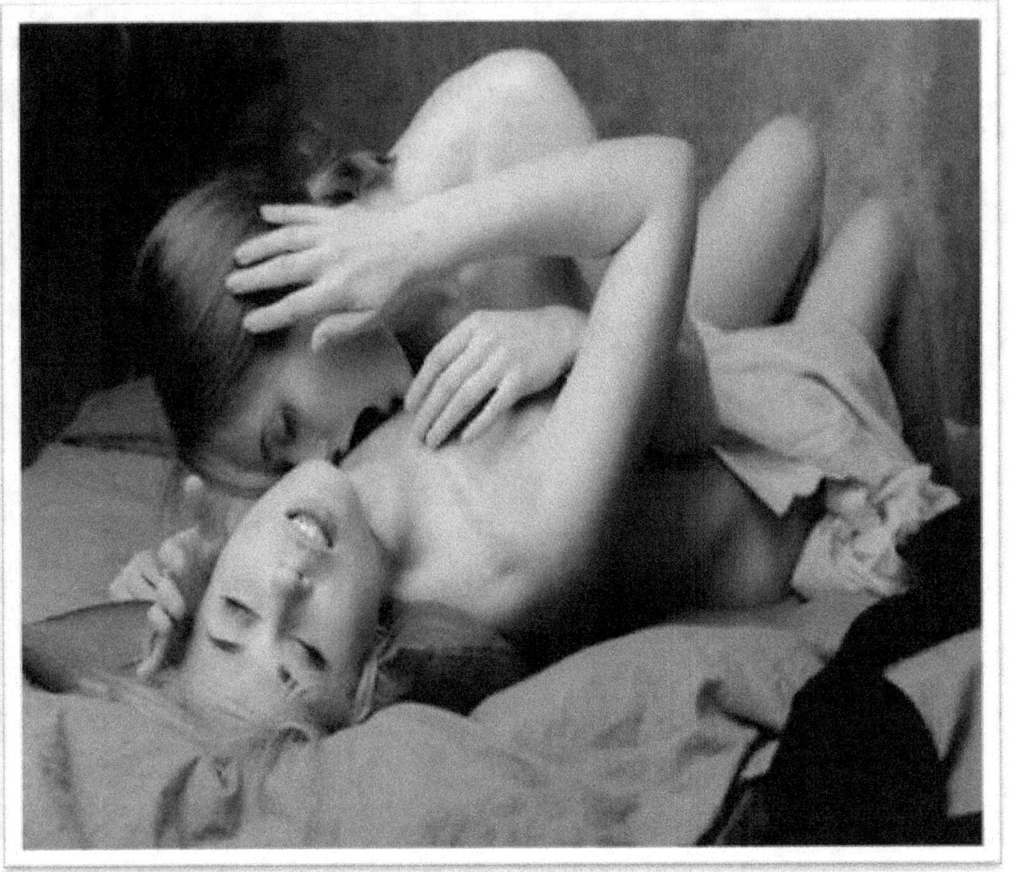

Chapter 2 The Importance of Intimacy

The word intimacy is frequently confused. Being intimate does not necessarily mean that you are having sex. There or a lot of sexual or physical acts that we participate in that actual house no intimacy at all. In this chapter, we are going to really get into the meat of what intimacy is. It affects us physically, mentally, and emotionally. When you have a good understanding of what intimacy is and what it means, your connection to your partner will be enhanced.

When you have a deep level of intimacy with another person, it also means that you know them on a different level than most others. It is something that takes an extended period of time. You won't become truly intimate with another person through a simple conversation or in spending a single day together. Intimacy will grow over time, as both people work to nurture their relationship. When both parties understand that mistakes happen and they forgive each other so that they can continue on and learn, true intimacy starts to develop.

For many people, intimacy can be frightening. This is because when you are intimate with someone, you have a deeper level of closeness than you do with others. Working through this fear leads to a strong and healthy relationship. Intimacy will develop and mature over the course of time by consistently revisiting it and facing the fears you have, together.

Intimacy involves a variety of different key aspects. Each one will play a role in deepening the connection between you and your partner. This connection will allow you to be truly intimate with another person. Let's take a look at the different pieces that one put together equal true intimacy.

The first component to true intimacy is allowing your partner to get to know you on the deepest level. You take the things that are held deep inside your soul and decide to share it with the person that you trust the most. Once you have shared these inner feelings, both parties will be able to see the value of the connection between the two of you. Additionally, the differences between you will be accepted, and you will work on coming to common ground easily.

Trusting someone with your innermost secrets is something that takes time. This is why intimacy is not developed at the very beginning of a relationship. You will need to spend time learning the more basic aspects of each other before either party is going to feel comfortable sharing more sensitive information. It is completely normal for true levels of intimacy to take time; in fact, it is basically a requirement. Most people are not apt to spill their innermost demons and desires. There is no concrete time frame in which true intimacy will be built; it is different for every couple.

Another factor that plays into true intimacy is acceptance. Sometimes, people get into a relationship because of the potential they see in another person. This is not a good thing. Sure, people change over the course of time, but their core nature tends to be the same. When you are going to try and truly be intimate with somebody, you need to understand that their flaws should be accepted, and they also need to accept yours. Trying to change a person in a fundamental way is never going to and up well.

We need to appreciate the uniqueness of our partner. Obviously, no two people are exactly the same. This should be celebrated; we should not look at it as a negative. Finding out the differences between you and your partner should be exciting. It should allow you to realize that there are points of view that are not your own, that are worth listening to. You can expand your thoughts and become better attuned to your emotions and yourself by listening to the ideas of the person you love.

Safety is another huge aspect of having the ability to be intimate with someone. When we are intimate, we are also very vulnerable. We need to trust that we are safe to be vulnerable with the person you are with. The ability to increase intimacy comes with knowing your partner supports your strengths, as well as your weaknesses.

Safety also comes from an understanding of your relationships. As a couple, you need to discuss the lines that can and cannot be crossed. By this, we mean things such as fidelity, finances, and where you are willing to go sexually. When these "rules" are defined, it leads to a feeling of security and understanding; in turn, both parties will be more apt to allow true intimacy to occur.

All relationships will come across bumps in the road. It is a normal and natural thing. When you are working toward true intimacy, you will work as a team. You will be compassionate when trying to solve a problem. Not only will you take your thoughts into consideration, but also your partner's. You should not be competing about who is right, rather working together to find a solution that is mutually beneficial.

The emotional connection with the person you are with will also play a big role in your intimacy level. When we are connected to someone on an emotional level, it makes growing intimacy much easier. You should be able to voice your opinions and concerns without worrying about the repercussions. In fact, voicing your opinion should deepen your connection; it should not hinder it.

Having an intimate relationship with someone will indeed affect you on a physical, emotional, and mental level. You will be sharing your whole self with someone. When you do this, you are allowing them to have an impact on you in every way. This means you need to be careful with whom you become intimate with. Later in this book, we will discuss intuition and compatibility; when we do, we will hit on this more.

Intimacy is something that needs to be cared for. It takes hard work and dedication. Relationships that last for a lifetime do so because they have been cared for. Intimacy should be a thing of focus from the beginning. You can't ignore intimacy without causing a detrimental impact on the relationship as a whole.

The choice of who you enter into a relationship with is exceptionally important. When we choose wisely in the beginning, it can set us up for success in terms of building a truly intimate relationship. You should never have to give up who you truly are to enter into a relationship. If you do, it is likely you are not making a wise decision. Obviously, every relationship requires some compromise, and you may even find yourself accommodating your partner from time to time. This is fine as long as you are not changing the core of your person.

Some signs that the person you are interested in or starting a relationship with is not right for you are:

- They blame you with no accountability for their own actions

- They try and keep you from your other friends

- They are not supportive of your thoughts and ideas

- They get mad with no understanding when you try and discuss serious topics

- They try and control the way you think and feel

- They ignore your wants, needs, and desires

- They misinterpret what you say and twist it to use it against you

- It feels impossible to express yourself truthfully

- You feel as if you are not being heard when you talk

- There is little or no room for compromise

These are only a few of the signs that you should look for when entering into a new relationship to choose whether or not it is one that will be healthy for you. Some things are more obvious to see than others. Taking the time to reflect on how your intended acts during serious situations can help you gain insight as to what a future with them may look like. Remember that while people change slightly throughout their lives, for the most part, they are who they are, and if they are right for you, you won't be thinking about their potential.

When we enter into a new relationship, we start to learn about the good and bad sides of a person. Showing yourself and exposing what you truly believe is a step in the right direction when trying to attain a truly intimate relationship. Know that when you express yourself in a raw way, the reaction may not be what you expect. Obviously, you want your partner to be understanding and supportive, but remember that it goes both ways. So, when they are expressing themselves, think about your reactions and how it is affecting the person you are developing feelings for.

Taking the time to look at your differences is very important. It can help you understand if the relationship is worth moving forward with. Having some beliefs that don't lineup is fine; however, if you are truly opposites, it wills likely lead to bigger problems down the road. Some differences can help us grow and evolve while others can be complete deal-breakers. Finding these things out, in the beginning, can help you avoid heartache and wasting your time.

Being emotionally mindful is another component in building intimacy with your partner. How we express, ourselves plays a role in helping or hurting the level of intimacy we experience. At one time or another, it is likely that you are going to have negative feelings toward your partner, this is normal, taking the time to consider how you should express them is really the important part.

You should trust your partner so that you can be honest with them, but you also need to be mindful of what you are saying. The words we use can cut deeply and cause the connection between the two of you to suffer. If you explode or become nasty because of heightened emotions, it could push your partner away and eventually lead to the demise of the relationship. So, be understanding and think before you speak to ensure that you and your lover stay closely connected and will be able to work through issues together.

Last, but not least, when working on nurturing your level of intimacy, work on being the best version of yourself that you can imagine. If you think that qualities like compassion, faithfulness, generosity, and understanding are important in a relationship, then work on being all of those things. No one is perfect, and we all have things to work on, but doing our best by someone else helps to make us worthy of intimacy. Do your best to be open and honest. Also, be willing to listen to their opinion and the feedback they give you on your thoughts.

Physical intimacy is not necessarily just sex; it is when we are affectionate with our partner. It includes things like holding hands, kissing, hugging, and cuddling. There should be a great physical connection when you are trying to achieve great levels of intimacy. When you are physical, in any way, with your partner, think about how it makes you feel. Are they good reactions or bad ones? By answering this simple question, it can become quite easy to see if this is the person you should be connecting with or not.

When we are intimate on a mental level, it means that we can easily express our thoughts and ideas about everything with another person. When we have the ability to truly share what is on our mind, it is going to enable us to become vulnerable with our partner. We trust them and, in turn, share all things with them. Their reactions are considerate, and we feel as if we have been heard. Connection on this mental level is a key element in true intimacy and a healthy relationship.

Emotional intimacy is probably one of the scariest forms for a lot of people. When you choose to be emotionally open, allowing your partner to see the lightest and darkest sides of you, it can be intimidating. However, when trust has been built, and lines of communication are open and honest, it really isn't as scary as many people think. True emotional intimacy will allow you to share your joy as well as your sorrow with another person. They will be there to support you whether you are feeling high on life or exceptionally low.

When you combine all three types of intimacy, you are looking at it in its most pure form. Reaching these levels of intimacy does not happen with every relationship, and it certainly does not happen overnight. In fact, it can only be accomplished in those relationships that are consistently worked on. When you find the person who you can open up to on every level, and that is willing to do the same with you, it is worth the effort. With continued effort, respect, openness, and caring, intimacy can truly solidify you as a couple and ensure your relationship is one that is healthy and happy in every area.

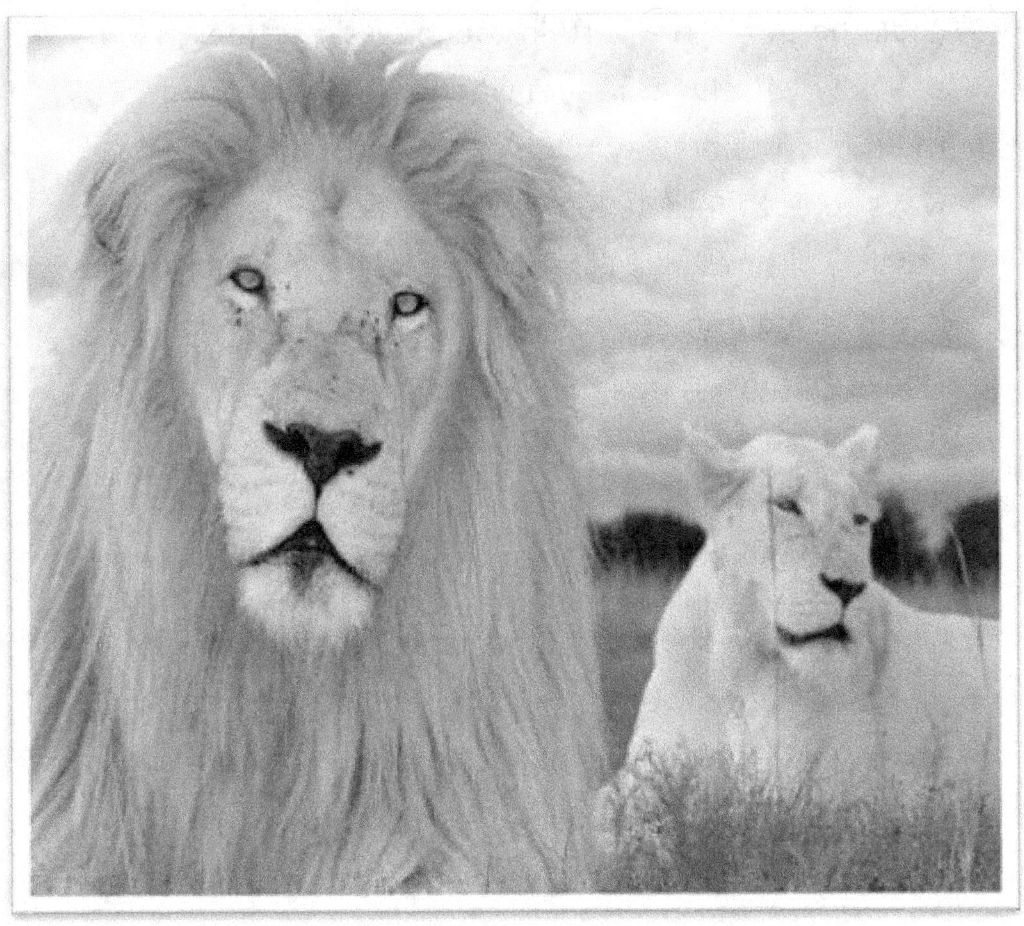

Chapter 3 Learning To Make Love (Practical Sex Advice)

Having sex for the first time can be an exciting and nervous experience full of anticipation. It involves a wide range of emotions. Once you become familiar with sex, even if on a basic level, you will begin to learn what brings you and your partner pleasure. It could be through a certain touch or sensation. Try to see how your lover reacts when you kiss or touch them in certain away. One of the most important ways to ease into sexual intimacy is through a gentle session of foreplay. This can be subtle, beginning with light kissing and touching, showing and exchanging signs of affection. During this phase, you may notice a decrease in anxiety and begin to experience signs of arousal. An erection is one of the initial signs in men, while women may feel their labia engorge and swell.

There may be slight wetness or moistening in the genital area, as well as heightened sensitivity to touch and sound. During this phase, the mutual attraction intensifies, which creates a transition to sex.

The Challenges of Sexual Education in Society

In many cultures and societies, sex education is considered taboo and avoided as much as possible. Even in countries where there is a more relaxed approach to the concept of sex and where it is introduced into the education system or discussed within the family, there still exists a gap between learning the fundamentals of biology and how to experience the pleasures of sexual activity. Sex education in most schools, for example, centers on the prevention of STIs (sexually transmitted infections), the concept of sexual arousal, and how the reproductive system works. In some progressive school systems, the curriculum has a broader spectrum of education to include all sexual orientations. These schools also have a more accepting approach to sexual and gender identity. However, there still exists a significant amount of resistance against a general openness to sexuality, and people are not generally taught how to enjoy and seek pleasure during sex.

Some family and marital arrangements have a heavy reliance on traditional practices that hold on to strict male and female roles. They place a more dominant role on men, with the expectation that women will always be sexually compliant and available even when there is no explicit consent. This power dynamic places men in a more commanding position where women's sexual needs and wants are suppressed.

On the other hand, men are expected to take on a traditional "leadership" role, which doesn't come with the goal of giving women pleasure or helping them achieve pleasure together as a couple. In relationships where there is both a lack of sexual education and mutual connection, sexual intimacy can be a major challenge, often done out of necessity and starting a family. Thus, it is less about pleasure and pleasing each other.

As some people break away from their traditional roles in marriage and intimate relationships, they realize there is much to learn from each other, especially on how to express their desires, bond with each other, and experience the joy of sex together.

While many people hold on to traditional views of marriage and sex, it is important to recognize the importance of learning the value of pleasure: how to please ourselves and our partners. This will only become easier for people once the stigma of sexual openness and communication fades away over time, allowing more discussion and direct communication about sex and how we can enjoy it.

Important Facts About Sex Everyone Should Know

Learning about sex goes beyond the basics of biology. It goes beyond responding to various cues and states of arousal. There are a lot of interesting facts to know about sex. If you are new to sex or less experienced, you will find that the early stages are a combination of learning from what you hear, read, and experience first-hand. If you are more knowledgeable than your partner, you can provide more guidance. However, care should always be taken so that both of you feel comfortable and willing to engage. The following important facts are vital and interesting, and they should be considered before you decide to engage with your partner.

1. Consent should be explicit.

When it comes to sex, a simple "Yes, I want to make love" is not always the way we consent or agree to have sex. When one partner initiates intimacy, the other may appear interested at first and then may hesitate later on. The reasons can vary, from changing their mind to simply not being interested in the moment. When there is the slightest doubt, it is important to establish whether consent is present, and make sure both of you are completely 100 percent willing without any reservations. There should be explicit consent, which means you and your partner should be fully in agreement and enthusiastic about it.

2. Sex is not going to be the same experience every time.

Some sessions will be groundbreaking and exciting, leaving you wanting more. On other occasions, sex is less than thrilling and may not bring both or either partner to orgasm. This can be a result of various things — e.g., personal trauma in life, stress from family or work, or simply not feeling completely engaged or aroused in the experience. This is perfectly normal. It would be unusual to have ideal sex each and every time, as this is unrealistic. Do not expect this to happen always. It is important to be realistic, and accept the fact that, on some occasions, the spark may not be present. Be patient, and you will find that the best experiences will return again.

3. Long sessions of sex do not equate to better quality, and short, quick sex does not always have to be negative either.

It really depends on the couple and the circumstances. For example, in the morning, a quick session of early sex may be brief but highly passionate and satisfying. In fact, both lovers may be familiar enough with each other to bring about orgasm within a short time span, and then they go their separate ways for work and other daily activities. A longer session in a rushed morning would not accommodate their schedule. On the other hand, a slower, deeper intimacy in the evening hours can be satisfying in a completely different way, allowing both partners to experience more of each other.

4. Erection does not happen instantly every time, and when it does, it may occur when it is least expected.

A man may find himself with an erection in the morning during a shower or as he's getting ready for breakfast. A woman, on the other hand, may feel aroused during regular activities, such as attending a conference or running errands. When sex is initiated, it may take time to achieve an erection and natural arousal, even where both lovers are ready and excited to begin.

5. Lubrication is good for everyone.

It is wonderful how our bodies can create our own wetness, though it is best to add a bit of natural lubricant to your sexual encounter to avoid dryness and irritation later. There are various brands to choose from. You can also choose a variety of flavors and/or scents. There is also a choice between a more sensitive and natural fluid versus a more standard one. Take time to shop around with your partner to determine which one works best for both of you.

6. Moving from one position to another during sex is not always a simple task.

It mainly depends on your flexibility. Try new poses or positions, and switch them up every now and then. Some moves are going to take some practice, even exercise, to get them just right. Some positions may require your partner to lend you a hand, or you may need to help them steady their balance or ease slowly into a new pose. It may not look and feel glamorous, but it will be fun just the same!

7. Using protection is important, and knowing how to use it is vital.

Condoms are the most commonly used and preferred method of birth control and protection against STIs (sexually transmitted diseases). They are important early in the relationship. However, learning how to use a condom for the first time can be frustrating, and it often causes friction if not lubricated well. Condoms are not all created equally. Some brands may boast high sensitivity, while others are more durable and already lubricated, making it easier to put on. To avoid potential breakage and to ensure your experience is not spoiled, make sure you have a few condoms handy, just in case. Read the instructions carefully and take it slowly at first until you become used to the procedure. Remember that your partner can be helpful and give you much-needed support and assistance to get your session underway. There are creative and fun ways of putting on a condom, and this can fit easily into foreplay, making the experience much more enjoyable.

8. Sex is good for your health, and it is a form of exercise.

The more often you engage, the more calories you will burn. It is great for the heart and your body in general. Sex itself is a euphoric experience, causing a release of endorphins in the body, which reduces the likelihood of depression, anxiety, and other disorders. The frequency of sex varies from one couple to another, and while it is often more often at the beginning of the relationship, a routine will eventually become established. Even if you are engaging twice a week, there are fantastic benefits to your health and well-being.

9. Smoking can have a negative impact on your sex life.

Not only is smoking bad for your health, but it is also associated with lower rates of arousal and a decline in the strength of an erection. It can also affect endurance, making it difficult for the smoker to last longer in the bedroom, especially where there are respiratory conditions involved. If you currently smoke, consider quitting or taking steps to decrease the amount you use, as this will make a major improvement over time.

10. Orgasm is not going to happen every time you have sex.

You can have a hot and passionate session with your partner and not achieve a climax. Likewise, your partner can experience the same; it happens for both men and women. It can cause feelings of disappointment and insecurity. It is normal for this to occur sometimes, even between health-loving couples.

11. The more you communicate, the better your sex life will be.

Many people avoid talking about certain topics, including sex and intimacy. When communication breaks down, it can lead to a lot of misunderstandings, hurt, and avoidance. Intimacy can eventually break down until it reaches the point where it is no longer a part of a couple's life. Once this happens, it can lead to marital or relationship breakdown as well. Keeping the conversation alive is the best way to enjoy all that your relationship can provide.

There are many other facts about sex that you can learn in a variety of ways. One of the best ways to get familiar with your body and to engage with your partner is through open dialogue and discussion about a variety of concerns, including your fantasies and desires (Gordon, 2018).

Five Uncommon Facts That Can Improve Your Sex Life

Getting comfortable with your partner will not only help improve your sex life but will also give you the confidence to ask questions and better understand how you can mutually pleasure each other. Exploring various techniques and ideas and having openness to doing so has a major impact on the success of your love life and how well it will develop over time. Couples who explore and communicate about sex without reservation tend to lead healthier, happier lives in general, not just in the bedroom.

There are a few unexpected ideas and facts that make a positive impact on your sex life. Some of these facts dispel myths about sex, giving us a different perspective on how to enjoy our love life. They also create a healthy outlook about sex and how we engage with our partner and ourselves.

1. *The most sexual part of our body is our brain.*

The onset of arousal and the creation of sexual fantasies begin here. It is our mind that plays the most significant role in how we experience lovemaking and how we connect with our partner. Our perception (the signals our body and mind process and send throughout our body during foreplay and sex) sets the stage for a spectacular series of sensations. Alternatively, when our thoughts or impressions about a specific scenario are negative, it affects our body's response. For example, if we feel hesitant about pursuing a specific technique with our partner or lack trust in them for some reason, even the usual pleasurable event of lovemaking can be unenjoyable. This is because your mind isn't completely involved or relaxed for the experience. When we feel connected in mind and body, sex only gets better over time.

2. *Women only orgasm 20 percent of the time during sex.*

This is usually because some men believe women can achieve climax with vaginal sex alone, whereas this is not often the case. In fact, most women need clitoral stimulation or oral sex to bring themselves to orgasm. In some positions, it is possible for both men and women to reach orgasm together, which can be incredibly pleasurable, though it can also take practice and time to achieve. It is also advantageous for couples to explore various forms of arousal, as well as positions that include oral sex. This will greatly increase the chances of orgasm for women and can help men as well.

3. Men also fake orgasms.

Women often admit to this, though men have been found to do this as well and often for the same reason: they want to please their partner or give the impression that they have been adequately satisfied. This may be a way for men to assure their partner that they are able to reach orgasm quickly and to convey confidence. For women, there are several reasons. Like men, they want to show their satisfaction or at least convince their partner of it. Faking an orgasm gives the other person the satisfaction of being able to bring their partner to climax and, therefore, boosts their ego or confidence. The problem with this technique is dishonesty. Faking an experience you should want to enjoy is not giving you any real pleasure, while at the same time, it gives your partner the wrong impression of what works for you.

4. Headaches and pain can often disappear or subside during sex.

The popular excuse for declining sex, "Not tonight, I have a headache," is usually joked about as a means to avoid intimacy or skip sex. In reality, such an excuse could mean something more, especially if it is a recurring phrase (or something similar). There may be a hidden discomfort associated with sex that your partner may not feel like explaining, though they may be more direct and open with patience and understanding. It is important to communicate to find out the real reasons for lack of intimacy and to gently approach the topic so as not to push or pressure your partner to explain everything, especially if there is (or are) reason(s) why they may not feel up to it (Hubby, 2017).

5. Many women masturbate, though they tend not to discuss it as freely or widely as men, mostly due to societal expectations and ideals.

Even where women have made great strides forward in freedom, including sexual expression and liberation, there are still items considered less favorable when broached by a woman than a man. Masturbation is one of these topics, as well as sex in general. However, this is changing, and women are becoming more vocal and expressive than ever. Masturbation, or self-pleasure, should never be a source of shame, whether you enjoy it for yourself or mutually with your partner (Carson, 2017).

Common Mistakes Men and Women Make During Sex

During the height of passion, where both lovers are completely mesmerized and connected, the slight error or misjudgment can thwart a good sexual experience completely. It happens even when we try our best, and knowing what can happen is one of the most important ways to avoid an embarrassing or uncomfortable situation that can impact the moment. Some mistakes we make are not sudden and unexpected; rather, they can become bad habits that repeat over time, dulling or killing the mood and atmosphere slowly over time or completely. Avoid this and other pitfalls to keep your sex life amazing and mind-blowing. The following are common errors people often commit during sex. These are also some of the worst culprits of a declining sex life:

1. Skipping foreplay completely.

This means no foreplay at all, not even for a minute. On average, foreplay occurs for about 10 or 15 minutes, and most men and women enjoy it more than they admit. Sometimes a quick session can mean less preparation time and more spontaneity, though this should not include leaving foreplay out of the picture completely. In fact, it should begin with foreplay and last at least for a couple of minutes. This stage is crucial in getting your partner aroused and ready for action. You will find that it benefits yourself as well, and the mutual affection grows together, setting the stage for a solid and enjoyable session of lovemaking, whether it is a quick play or a long and passionate session.

2. Poor hygiene.

This is a complete turn-off and can stop intimacy in its tracks. A little body odor or sweat after a trip to the gym or long cycling trip is natural and can actually be a turn-on, though a lack of proper hygiene on a recurring basis will often stop sexual attraction, especially if it becomes a habit. Taking good care of your body and how you treat yourself does not need to include fancy perfumes and body sprays. Your natural scent is a part of the attraction, and with proper hygiene, your sex life will only get better.

3. Focusing on perfection.

Do not look in the mirror during sex and expect your body and your partner's to resemble a glamorous sex scene on television or film. You are not having sex to impress but to have fun and enjoy intimacy with your partner. Focusing too much on how to look better and appeal more to your partner may seem reasonable; we all want to look our best and get the most out of lovemaking. However, it can become unreasonably obsessive. Some people become so saturated in the way they look, even when their partner is happy with them as they are, that the pursuit of perfection can actually harm their marriage and sexual relations. Obsessing too much on your flaws takes the focus away from your partner and enjoying each other.

4. Talking about ex-partners or ex-spouses.

At some point in a relationship, the subject will arise, and that is expected. However, it should not become a focal part of a conversation, especially where sex is involved. It is one of the top ways to turn off your partner and disengage. When you or your partner are in a heightened state of arousal, there's nothing worse than hearing about someone's ex-partner and how they employed certain sexual techniques in the bedroom. This will only give the impression that you are not interested in your partner, even where this is not the case at all. It can appear that by bringing up your ex, you are making a comparison between them, which can cause insecurity, even jealousy. Always choose your words carefully, and avoid discussion about past lovers, as they are no longer relevant.

5. Talking too much during sex.

This can be a turn-off, unless it is part of the act, such as sweet whispers and/or dirty talking, which can be deeply arousing and fun. Talking about unrelated matters, such as work, other people, and household matters, can dull the experience during sex. This can happen if at least one partner becomes bored, and this can occur when sexual intimacy becomes routine or in a rut and no longer the fun, eventful activity it once was. If this becomes an issue, make it a point to try new and exciting positions. Play scenarios and techniques, many of which are covered in this book!

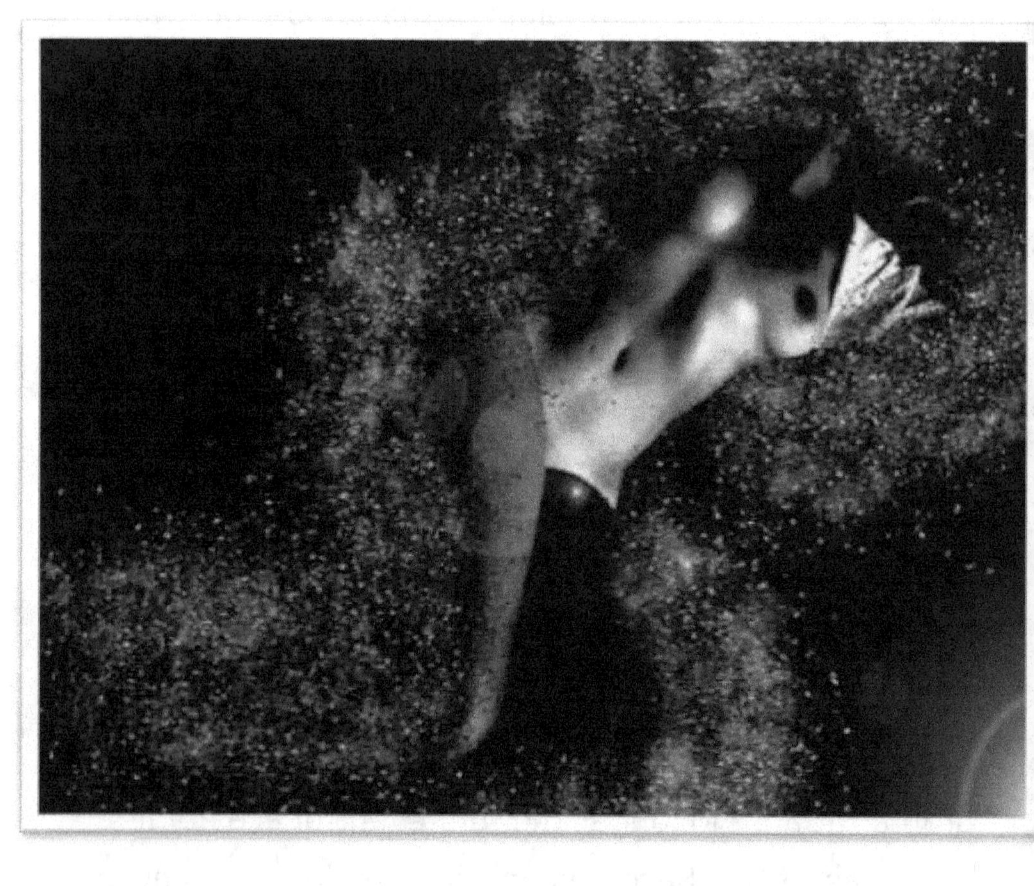

Chapter 4 Orgasm

The orgasm is the culmination of a sexual relationship, a climax that produces a pleasant feeling of a sudden release of accumulated tension from the moment when the excitement phase begins. It is at that moment that a series of intense muscle spasms are generated that is highly pleasing, which helps the release of endorphins that occurs simultaneously.

Women experience orgasm in different ways, but usually, this is characterized by the fact that the acceleration of heart rate, breathing, and blood pressure reach their highest level and the vagina, uterus, anus, and muscles Pelvic bones contract between five and ten times at intervals of less than one second. However, some women may feel orgasm throughout their body and even multiple orgasms.

In the case of men, we must bear in mind that ejaculation and orgasm are not the same. You can ejaculate without experiencing orgasm. As in women, with orgasm, heart rate, breathing, and blood pressure are accelerated to the maximum, and muscle contractions occur in the pelvic area, as well as the prostate and seminal vesicles to produce the expulsion of the semen.

The orgasm lasts only a few moments and then enters what is known as the resolution phase in which there is a general relaxation of the whole body, normalization of blood circulation and breathing, and with it a feeling of great placidity, tiredness, and even drowsiness.

The lack of control over ejaculation, as in the case of premature ejaculation, can make a man unable to reach orgasm. Similarly, many women confess not to reach it regularly and even never (anorgasmia). It is very important that the couple talks about it because experimentation and information can improve their sexual practice and learn to control ejaculation in the case of men and enhance their excitement in the woman. Couples therapy can be a good option to solve this sexual dysfunction.

How Are Male And Female Orgasms Different?

The female orgasm

Contractions start at 0.8-second intervals and their number can vary greatly, decreasing after intensity, duration, and frequency. More than a localized response in the pelvis, it is a total response of the organism. Imagination is directly related to orgasm, the brain has a lot to do with it. With the penetration, the entire vulvar pyramid is mobilized synchronously and the G-spot and the clitoris are stimulated. Every woman has the physical ability to experience orgasms.

These are the symptoms of female orgasm :

- Greater increase in heart rate.
- Increase in breathing
- Increase in blood pressure.
- The subjective sensation of the explosion of pleasure.
- Contraction of the uterus.

Contraction of the orgasmic platform.

After the orgasm, there would be a recovery in the woman prior to the excitement. Although if it is restimulated before the sexual tension decreases, the woman is able to present several successive orgasms.

The Female Orgasm: Keys To Reach It

The female orgasm is not only achieved through penetration. It is highly recommended to explore the female body to discover erogenous zones that facilitate the task. In the case of sexual intercourse, preliminaries, oral sex, and other pleasurable practices can be the perfect vehicle to achieve an unforgettable orgasm. Meanwhile, it is also essential:

- That your partner knows how to "work" better to "play" and experience things with you

to know oneself through self-exploration. So, if you want to enjoy your body and your areas of pleasure, try one of these useful toys.

1. Physical manifestations of female orgasm

During orgasm:

- the clitoris retracts,
- the vagina, the perineum and the uterus contract due to shaking
- the nipples harden
- the heart accelerates

the blood vessels dilate.

Everything is stimulated during this supreme pleasure with which women (and men, in their case) go mad. And it is normal because the orgasm involves secretion of endorphins, the molecule of happiness, which provides a feeling of unequaled well-being.

2. *How to achieve a female orgasm*

In general, most women achieve orgasm when they stimulate sexual areas alone or in pairs:

- Preliminary caresses: activate your brain preparing for the moment of intercourse. These movements increase the pleasure much more and reach orgasm before.
- cunnilingus: is one of the techniques that most excites women and that will favor that if you have anorgasmia you can get to reach orgasm.
- masturbation: whether you do it yourself or your partner will get the genital area excited more easily.

penetration: through the penis the woman also reach orgasm. It is one of the most essential parts that lead us to intercourse, to the female orgasm, and also to the ejaculation of man.

But the best way to reach orgasm knows the body of one. We have different erogenous points that are able to make us feel in the seventh heaven, but you have to find them!

The solution: start in the discovery of the body:

- alone or as a couple,
- with sexual toys

without them, to detect the most moving areas.

3. Different female orgasms

Vaginal orgasm: is achieved by stimulation of the Gräfenberg point or more commonly called "G-spot", located about 4 cm from the entrance of the vagina. It has a ball shape of less than one centimeter and increases in size with stimulation. It is located next to the bladder so it is not strange that after a vaginal female orgasm we feel like going to the bathroom. To sensitize, stimulate it regularly with gentle and repeated pressures with the point of the finger or with the help of a sex toy. Try these toys if you want to get an incredible vaginal orgasm:

- Massager vibrator with 30 different modes.
- Chinese vibrating silicone balls with remote control .

Vibrator with heat effect for women .

Clitoral orgasm : is achieved by stimulation of the clitoris. That is a small button located between the lips, anterior to the vagina. It is accessed very easily. It is very sensitive. You can reach orgasm with delicate caresses. Here we leave you a few positions that will facilitate the pleasant task. These are the best sex toys to stimulate the clitoris:

- Satisfier Pro, clitoral sniffer.
- Clitoral massager with cunnilingus effect.

Vibrator clitoris massager.

4. The female orgasm, in figures

Clitorian orgasm: according to a study 95% of women come to him through masturbation and less than half, 45% share it with the male penis.

The vaginal orgasm: there are few women who manage to reach this orgasm. Only 30% have the pleasure of experiencing such pleasure. Although we all have a G-spot, we have to get "wake up" with multiple movements in this area. For this, there are positions that favor it: the missionary, with the legs of the woman on the back of the man or the greyhound, with which a deep penetration is facilitated.

5. *Female multiorgasm is possible*

Although for some it is only a fantasy, the truth is that multiorgasm exists and is easier to achieve than it seems. The key is in:

- know your own body,
- know what is possible
- put our mind on it,
- lengthen the sexual climax (many times we do not achieve it because our partner lasts less than we would like),
- go changing stimuli and erogenous zones

choose postures that really work with us

The Male Orgasm

There are between 3 and 10 contractions with an interval of 8 tenths of a second between each one, depending on how intense the response is. This means that an orgasm lasts on average between 4 and 8 seconds. Man experiences this physiological reaction as a wave of pleasurable sensations.

These are the symptoms of male orgasm :

- Greater increase in heart rate.
- Increase in breathing

- Increase in blood pressure.
- The subjective sensation of the explosion of pleasure.
- Contraction of the penis, urethra, and sphincter.

Expulsion of semen abroad.

After the orgasm, in man, there would be the recovery of the state prior to the excitement and the refractory period would begin, by which the man will not be aroused again after some time, something that can vary according to each person.

The Male Orgasm: Keys to Reach It

Orgasms during sex are better than during masturbation.
Orgasms during sex are significantly better than those experienced in solitude through masturbation. The transcendence of orgasms through sexual intercourse is because the man's body releases 400 times more prolactin than when he masturbates, for which several studies have shown that having low prolactin levels affects the sexual health of men and can lead to erectile dysfunction.

Ejaculating usually reduces the risk of cancer

The male orgasm has valuable potential to fight cancer. Men who ejaculated more frequently (about 21 times a month) reduced their risk of prostate cancer by 20 %. This benefit is since during the orgasm, different hormones are released, such as oxytocin (known as lowering blood pressure, for example).

Sperm is better in the morning.

 Orgasms during sex are significantly better than those experienced in solitude through masturbation. The transcendence of orgasms through sexual intercourse is because the man's body releases 400 times more prolactin than when he masturbates, for which several studies have shown that having low prolactin levels affects the sexual health of men and can lead to erectile dysfunction.

Is there a "dry" orgasm?

Yes. The dry orgasm or retrograde orgasm occurs when the man reaches the sexual climax but without ejaculation since the semen instead of being expelled by the penis stays inside the bladder due to a malfunction of the muscle. This type of orgasm is more common among preadolescent children than in adults. Retrograde ejaculation does not prevent achieving an erection or having an orgasm. The cause of dry orgasm in adults can come from several factors: side effects of some medications for the prostate or blood pressure, depression, surgery in the bladder or prostate or year in the nerves caused by multiple sclerosis or diabetes.

The male and female orgasms are more similar than it seems

Despite the difference in orgasm between men and women, there is no variation between the duration and intensity of orgasm concerning sex. What does offer opposition is that the orgasms are different in each person and can be divided into two main types: the usual orgasm, the most common, consisting of about 6-15 high-intensity contractions for about 20-30 seconds or orgasm prolonged, in which regular contractions are experienced after the initial orgasm, which can last between 30 and 90 seconds.

Male ejaculation is as fast as ...

The average speed of a man's ejaculation is 45 kilometers per hour. Taking into account that Usain Bolt runner holds the record of 44.72 kilometers per hour, the rate of ejaculation is faster than the fastest man on the face of the Earth.

Men can have multiple orgasms

Most men who can achieve multiple orgasms need at least a refractory period of 30 minutes between each sexual activity. However, some men can reach orgasm without ejaculation, as in the case of dry orgasm. According to experts, the key to achieving this is training.

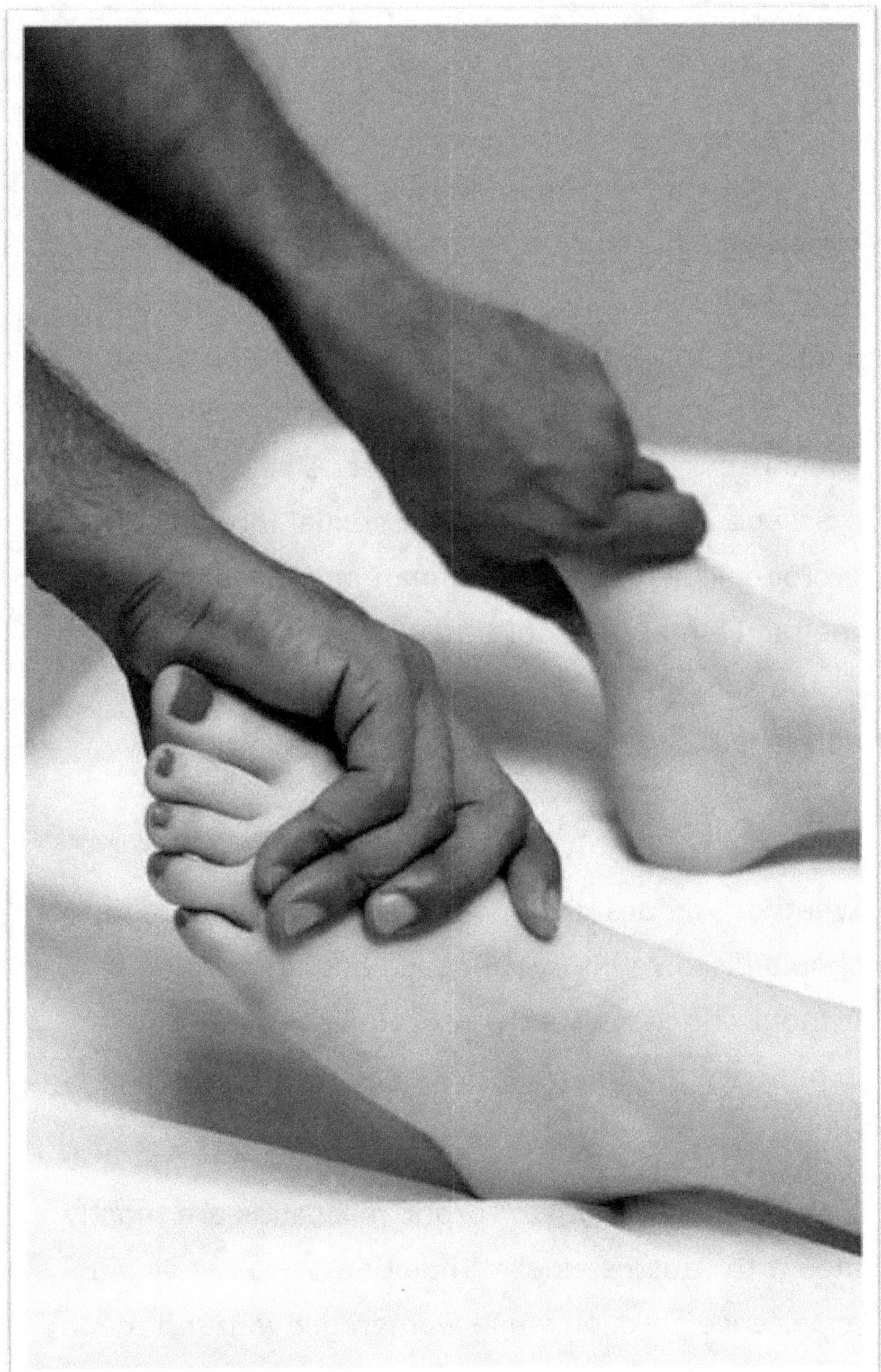

Chapter 5 Practical An Erotic Massage Advice

Our bodies have tremendous capabilities to experience pleasure through the five ordinary senses. Above all, the sense of touch is explored to attain exquisite joy, especially in intimacy. If you are in a loving relationship, erotic massage is a means you could use to stimulate each other. Chiefly, touch, and massage is a powerful tool for sexual foreplay. The erotogenic aspect of the human body aids in receiving the tactile massages of desire, love, and tenderness. At the same time, the soul and emotions become nourished.

Benefits of Erotic Massage

Whether you are giving or receiving the massage, you should dissolve into your space and learn to do it without criticism. That way, you rest assured to experience the following benefits from the feeling of touch.

1.   *Facilitates orgasm:* Erotic massages are mostly meant to cause sexual stimulation. As a result, men experience erection while women get wet and moody.

These are body responses to allow for perfect intercourse.

2.   *Enhances Relationships:* If you would like to see your relationship blossom, then you need to incorporate erotic massage in your foreplay. The practice requires you to be emotionally open and conscious. Consequently, you develop a mutual connection that promotes your relationship.

3.   *Relieves anxiety:* Your body has endorphin that allows muscle relaxation after the massage. The relaxation helps reduce stress and anxiety, making it a perfect after-work must do.

4.   *Fights Inflammation*: Erotic massage is ideal in improving your muscle health and joints. It relaxes and stimulates aching and overworked muscles. Your body becomes flexible and refreshed to proceed with the daily routine.

5.   *Tone the Skin*: Erotic massage cleanses your skin by rubbing it gently and unblocking pores. You remain clean as you wipe unwanted layers. Incorporation of massage oil plays a significant role in reviving the natural tone of your skin.

6. *Improves Blood Circulation*: During the massage, the blood flows throughout the body to meet the threshold for sexual stimulation. The heart pumps in moderation as the relaxation enhances circulation.

7. *Relaxes Muscles*: As you receive the message, your body experiences gentle and frequent muscle contractions. The process of compressing the muscles is vital in correcting rigid tendons.

8. *Regulates Hormones*: Massages are known to cause pleasure and stimulation. Specifically, erotic massage helps in boosting your moods and urge. Further, the massage improves your immune system, thus improving the ability to fight infections.

What You Need

Before indulging in the act itself, you should first recall a previous massage session. Create an atmosphere that surpasses what you experienced. In most cases, couples would need to take a warm shower to help relax muscles. The following preparations are crucial in making your room a haven of seduction.

- *Get Rid of Distractions:* The most crucial thing about erotic massage is that it works miracles in a quiet and peaceful place. Therefore, you should settle and focused on the activity while avoiding interruptions. Notably, the requirement includes all sorts of distractions, whether physical or psychological.

- *Lighting:* Erotic massage is perfect when done in relatively dim light to create an ethereal atmosphere. For that reason, you should set sources of dim light such as candles to make it warm and cozy. You should apply proper caution as you may be prone to burns.

- *Fragrance:* Scents play a significant role in influencing a person's moods and memories. The application of essential oils and incense sticks provide a therapeutic and pleasant fragrance.

- *Music:* Music is also an important part, especially if it is suitable for erotic massage. It should create a spa atmosphere and should even flow in a sexual and soothing mood.

- *Temperature:* While most couples may prefer a naked erotic massage, the room temperature should be regulated accordingly. You may use a warm sheet to keep your partner comfortable during the massage. Room temperature would be preferable but might be subject to change depending on your adaptation.

How Is It Done?

You should start with gentle touches as you build comfort and confidence with the process. Your partner should help you in deciding whether to start with the hands or feet. The fact that sensual massage acts as foreplay means that you should feel free to seduce your partner. Therefore, you are required to increase physical contact for great feelings of intimacy. Feel free to massage the whole body and pay close attention to nerve endings. Application of techniques serves as a powerful gift that is pleasurable, intimate, and demonstrates selflessness.

Types of Erotic Massage

In addition to releasing stress and tension, erotic massage can also help you focus on the pleasurable sensation. In most cases, these forms of massage end up in ejaculation or orgasms.

1.   *Soapy Massage*: It starts in the shower when naked couples rub soap onto one another. The soap

aids in giving a smooth massage as well as cleaning them for further massage or sex.

2. *Duo Massage*: It mostly involves two people giving and receiving luxurious massage. Both the giver and the receiver apply oil on their bodies for a perfect body to body massage.

3. *Prostate Massage*: This form of massage aims at stimulating the prostate glands mostly believed to be a man's emotional, sacred, and sexual spot. Stimulated prostate releases psychological and physical pressure that creates an intense experience.

4. *Lingam Massage*: It involves honoring the stimulation and sensations of the penis through massage. It includes gentle touches on the testicles, shaft, and the perineum. It is meant to create sensual stimulation from a thorough genital massage.

5. *Yoni Massage*: Such as the lingam, Yoni involves loving, respecting, and honoring vaginal stimulation through massage. A relaxed yoni massage helps create acceptance of the sexual feelings experienced. This type of erotic massage is beneficial, especially if you want to release sexual issues such as sexual pain

and anorgasmia. It is known to build trust and respect in relationships.

Erotic massage is vital in your foreplay, for it allows you to influence your partner's sexual desires. You develop a mutual concept when you exercise different forms of erotic massage. However, you should be careful and deliberate not to mistake a tickle for a massage.

Learning to Make Love

As a couple, you may have similar desires and wants, but the sequence required may differ. In most cases, men are known to take less time to achieve sexual stimulation as compared to women. If you are inexperienced in making love or seem to be unskilled, you need to understand what making love entails. How you approach your partner as well as the way you handle the situation plays a significant role in achieving orgasm. It would be advisable to research what you could be doing wrong if your partner complains of sexual dissatisfaction. Similarly, you could explore additional information on ways to make your lovemaking more lively and enjoyable. The following detailed steps to step guide will help you on how you could be a pro in making love.

1.   *Nurture your self-esteem*: Appreciating your personality and character is the initial point where you develop an excellent reflection about yourself. You should explore your thoughts honestly and openly to identify the aspect that could be hindering you from attaining your full potential. Similarly, you realize your strengths and weaknesses are making it easier to gauge your potential and select tasks. This way, you will be able to relieve yourself of the things that cannot be changed as well as those that are from the past. Notably, this process requires ample time to internalize the steps you need to take to get rid of negative interactions that always drag you behind. It may even entail adjusting your environment and finding time to do what you enjoy. The critical aspect of improving your self-esteem is embracing change. As it may be difficult in the initial stage, you need to be patient and perseverant to achieve the benefits of being a confident, healthier, and happier person.

2.   *Improve Your Lifestyle*: After developing high self-esteem and making the right moves to understand yourself, you remain qualified to build a healthy love

life. As you explore those various aspects that will offer guidance on your dating life, you need to keep on developing your confidence and selecting a reasonable target. You will realize that making love involves flirting, teasing, and providing compliments as you aim to take your partner to the bed. Developing your intimacy skills will play a vital role in arousing your mind, which then makes you anticipate a gentle touch and intimacy. Besides, you should note that how you present yourself is an excellent determinant of the partner you win and their perception about you. Therefore, you must get a life and begin to make natural moves of seduction and arousal.

3. *Understand What It Is to Make Love*: This is an essential part of making love for you might mistake making love for sex. If you do not see any difference, then you might not have experienced it. Sex is familiar to everyone and involves biomechanical and instinctive intercourse. On the contrary, lovemaking is all about the art of sensual and slow romance. Lovemaking is meant to create a connection between partners. The motivation for lovemaking differs from that of sex. Lovemaking is a complex act of

expressing love and satisfying your partner. It is an activity where your body, soul, and mind are equally involved in getting to each other's heart. The openness associated with lovemaking allows all forms of communication, leaving no room for wandering. Lovemaking starts long before intercourse and may continue after that. For that reason, you should consider lovemaking as an emotional activity but not just undressing and romping on the bed.

4.   *Pick Perfect Location*: Lovemaking should happen in a place where you feel comfortable and undistracted. Therefore, you should ensure that the site you choose for lovemaking is romantic. If you would like to make it more personal, you could select a comfortable room in your house where you are aware of the environment. Be creative while choosing your location and consider aspects such as weather and your partner's preference. Also, the temperature of your preferred location should be in line with the activity ahead as too warm or cold could make it a mess. Remember to put away all forms of distractions to avoid losing the true meaning of making love.

5.   *Set The Mood*: If it is your first time to make love, you need to be sure and comfortable about what you

are about to do. Ensure that you are aware of what is about to happen and decide on what outcomes you expect. Similarly, make the ambiance conducive and appropriate for lovemaking. When you are in for it avoid being silly or making tasteless jokes thinking that your partner likes it. Instead, settle on a romantic atmosphere where everything you do aims at soothing them and causing sexual stimulation. With this course, your partner will feel appreciated, safe, and cherished through cuddling and gentle touches. Setting the mood may also involve sexy details such as dirty words, music, movies, dim light, and lingerie. When the attitude is right, you will tell from the responses you get from your partner as well as your body reaction.

6.   *Focus on Foreplay*: It is worth noting that lovemaking starts way before sex hence the importance of engaging in stimulating foreplay. It is the best moment to put off the fears and doubts about yourself or your partner. Besides, foreplay prepares your bodies for sex, especially when done accordingly. Notably, men may experience different feelings during foreplay, and it is essential to ensure that you please your partner by customizing various

forms of foreplay. Most women like it when their partners take time during foreplay and incorporate stimulating touches. You should not be in a hurry or skip foreplay for it is pleasurable and makes your partner submit unconditionally. Ensure you observe your partner's reaction to the different techniques you apply so as not to hurt or annoy them. Making love aims at pleasing your partner as you enjoy too. Be selfless and make them feel pampered, unique, and loved. The selflessness reciprocates, and you should rest assured that it creates a memorable event for both of you.

7.   *Pick Positions to Achieve Intimacy*: Making love involves openness and finding ways to connect with your partner. The connection can be achieved physically, spiritually, and emotionally. Notably, intimacy is performed depending on the level of contact your body is having with that of your partner. Therefore, you should ensure that your body is in better positions and preferably on face-to-face posture. There are various sex positions that you could apply to please your partner and have the best of experiences in intimacy. Sex positions make it easier to communicate while exploring each other's

bodies. As you will find from the next chapter, there are benefits associated with each sex positions, and it would be advisable to find a collection that best works for you. For example, spooning and missionary positions are recommendable for they allow full-body contact thus achieving intimacy. Avoid distracting and challenging positions, especially on your initial dates.

8.   *Feedback*: Most couples find it hard to share their experiences after sex. It proves challenging for men to provide feedback to women on their performance. However, you should understand that telling each other how you feel could make a significant difference in your intimate life. Besides, this form of communication helps you establish a deep connection. When partners provide positive feedback, they nurture their confidence towards each other, thus promoting perfection and further exploration. Similarly, correcting each other makes you skillful and well cognitive of your partner's hidden treasures. Lovemaking does not end immediately after sex, and that is why you should continue cuddling after sex to extend intimacy and show appreciation.

Making love is experienced after your mind and body develop feelings and intimate emotions. It is an act

that brings you closer to your partner, both
emotionally and physically.

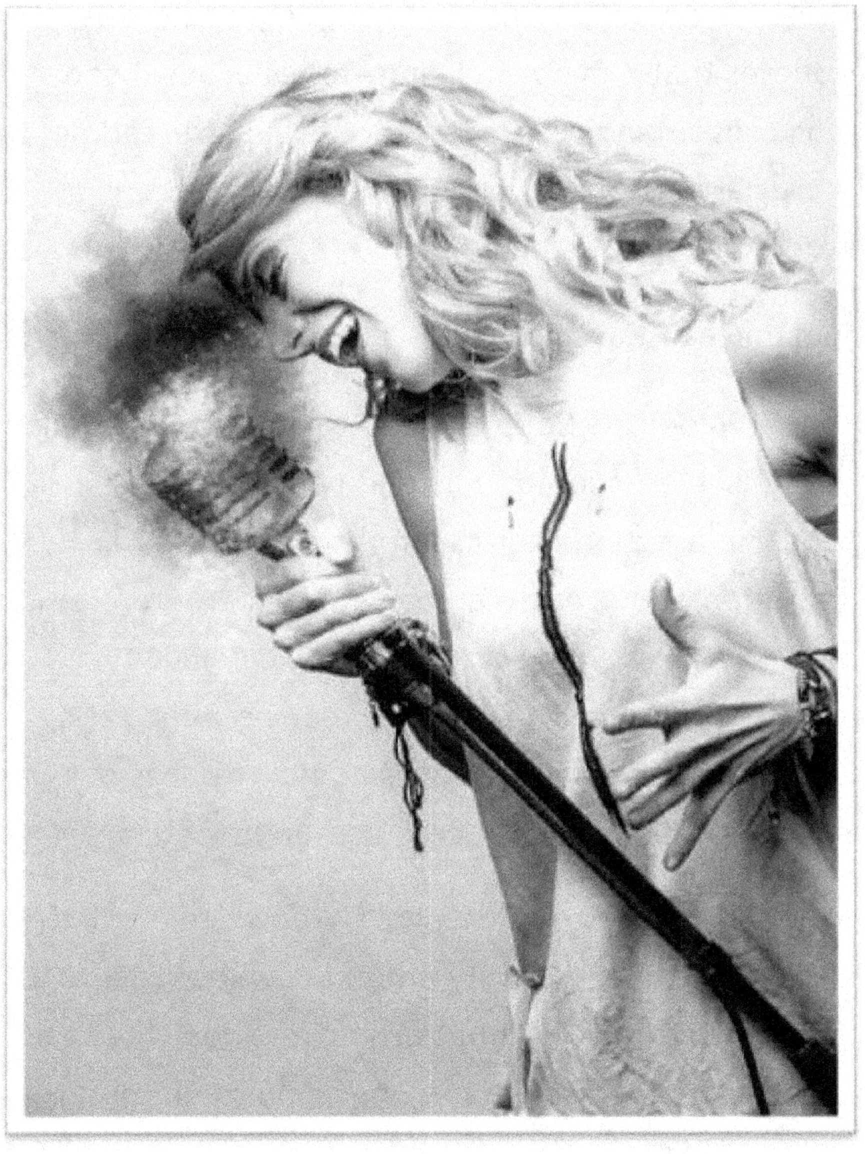

Chapter 6 Foreplay (Oral Sex Techniques, Use Only Your Hands)

Foreplay is an activity at the beginning of a sexual encounter that aims at building sexual arousal and brings orgasm in preparation for sexual intercourse. It is a crucial part of sexual experience and acts as a determinant of satisfaction.

Importance of Foreplay

- Biological: Couples need to indulge in foreplay for it causes erection of both the penis and the clitoris. An erection is crucial for it enhances penetration and orgasm among women. Therefore, it creates the best conditions for biological activity. Besides, foreplay elicits wetness making penetration easier for the couples. Lack of vaginal wetness is associated with painful intercourse and bleeding.

- Psychological: Foreplay is known to instill a feeling of care and security among couples. Failure to make foreplay makes your partner feel neglected and denied emotional assurance. The concern of your partner's feeling before sex serves as an indicator that you are not in for selfish gains but mutual pleasure.

Types of Foreplay

Foreplay is the ultimate time to build tension and sexual chemistry between partners. If you lack mind-blowing sex, you should focus on foreplay. Notably, sex is more realistic and complex than what television and movies show. For that reason, when you intimately touch, smell, hear, and taste your partner, they would argue it as better than penetration.

The following are types of foreplay that you should work before sex.

1.   Sexy Materials: You could practice foreplay at any time and manner. You do not have to be naked to engage in foreplay. When at home or work you may watch a sexy movie or read sexy materials. These materials could help you maintain orgasm for hours.

2.   Undressing: If you usually take off your clothes before sex, then you might be missing a lot of foreplay. Having your fingers hold your partner's outfits and graze on their body as you undress them is highly stimulating and arousing. Depending on how sensitive they are, you might witness them getting goosebumps.

3.   Vagina stroking: It involves how you put your hands down there and caressing on her pants and panties. Light strokes on the region make her wet and stimulated for sex.

4.   Kisses and caressing: Though kisses do not lead to sex, most sexual activities involve kisses and touching. As part of foreplay, kisses should start slow and intensify gradually. Kisses on the neck and boobs are most arousing for women.

5.   Boob Action: Teases made on their breasts arouse women. Therefore, you should suck, kiss and rub them, taking advantage of the sensitive nerve ending in the nipples. The foreplay should be done with moderation to avoid hurting your partner.

6.   Dry Hump: It involves gently grinding on your partner. It can happen when naked to show how moody you are. The foreplay plays a significant role in heating the moment for intercourse.

7.   Breathing: Yes, you are right; your breath arouses and stimulates your partner, especially when done on sensitive areas such as genitals and neck. In this case, bad breath would be counterproductive.

8.   Hands-On: Your hands are a piece of efficient equipment when it comes to foreplay. You should use them to grab your partner's breasts, rub their hair, and thighs. In short, use your hands to explore your partner's body unless they say no.

9.   Oral: If you are okay in giving oral, you should incorporate it into your foreplay routine. Be a little bit gentle by teasing, sucking, and licking the clitoris and allowing time.

10. Labia love: As a highly ignored part, labia have numerous nerve endings that are perfect for arousal and stimulation. You can massage them slowly or hold them gently between fingers.

11. Ass: If you and your partner are into stimulation through the anus, then you should try it out effectively. The most ignored nerve endings in the anus cause sexual stimulation, especially if gently licked.

12. Multitask: You may incorporate all of these techniques and concurrently make different moves. With the perfect combination, you make your partner fantasized with enjoyable sexual stimulation

How Do I Give Mind-Blowing Foreplay?

The list of foreplay techniques proves that the activity is a real deal when it comes to sexual arousal. Similarly, mastering the best and most applicable to your partner is a significant step towards sexual satisfaction. You may learn the best technique but wrong application of foreplay may be counterproductive to both partners. For that reason, it is advisable to understand the following steps when going for foreplay.

•   Relax: Although partners have different timeframes to achieve orgasm, it may take about 3 minutes and twenty minutes for men and women respectively. So you should take your time and allow time to climax.

•   Make it gradual: You should start the foreplay with the areas away from the genitals with slow stimulation. With hot breaths, kisses, stroking, you are sure to achieve orgasm once you hit the spot.

•   Caress gently: You should make progressive touches on the less apparent spots of your partner's body, such as buttocks and inner thighs. You should delight the nipples with light feathery touches. In the same way, you should gradually approach the genitals from the outer layers as you move inner.

•   Adjust Stimulation: An ongoing touch on nerve endings reduces their sensitivity. Therefore, you should vary strokes from light to strong and move from one spot to another.

•   Seek Feedback: Most partners feel shy, asking for what they want in foreplay. However, they appreciate it when asked if they enjoy the foreplay. With questions like "How does it feel?" there is good communication and willingness to please a partner. The practice promotes intimacy and enjoyable sex.

•   Practice: You should indulge in foreplay without penetration to know your partner and lead them to repeat orgasms. Continued engagement in other forms of sexual interaction acts as an eye-opener in your sexual horizons.

Sex may hurt if your partner is not ready. Foreplay acts as a preparation for enjoyable sexual intercourse. Ensure that you apply the foreplay that best fits you to avoid accidents and incidents.

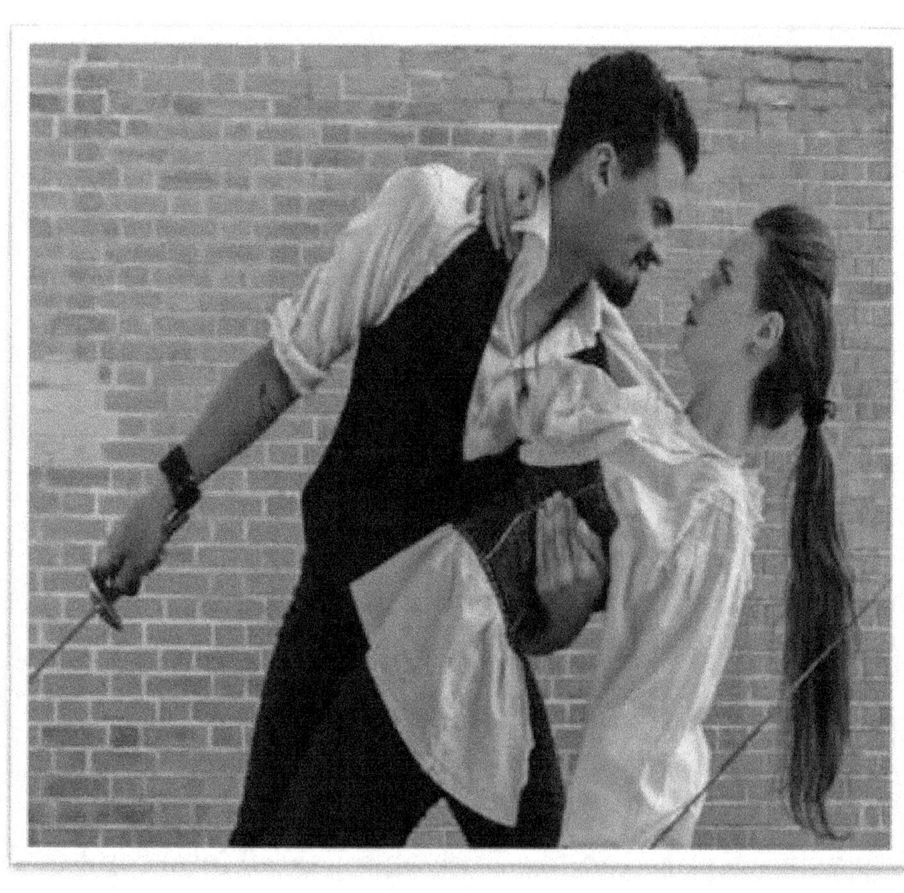

Chapter 7 Beginners Positions (Man On Top, Woman On Top)

Man On Top

Man on top is not the dominance of man to woman, but an equitable way of pleasure for both partners. It allows them constant eye contact and easy access to kissing, licking bodies and sucking boobs. Plus, it is quite relaxing and enjoyable to put the man on control and lie down, being on top of her and going deep inside, spicing the experience of both partners up. It allows the man to adjust his body towards her navel so that his penis gets deeper and deeper into the vagina, proving a strong stimulation and a rubbing experience to the inner lips of the vagina. This could be varied by small movements, like straightening the legs and allowing him to shallow or bending knees by either of the partners. Or even by allowing the male to stay on feet and go straight and deep with friction into the vagina. Many variations are possible with enormous hidden joys. Variations will crave both partners to indulge deep into sex and experience unforgettable joys.

Missionary

This sex position, famously known as missionary, is one of the most desirous situations to get the most out of sex and guarantee satisfaction for you and your lady. It allows both male and female counterparts to lie down, with the man on top and full exposure of the figure. Bodies are joined tightly, providing sensible, emotional and feeling exposure, with male's back hold tightly by female counterpart and legs in between the wide opened legs of the female partner. It enthusiasts to go deeper inside of the vagina with an elegant face, lips, neck, and breasts kissing due to the full exposure of figure, not only for the male but also for the female, gifting an adventurous climbing with deep penetration. This is one of the few positions that guarantee frictionless and thorough penis inclusion inside of the vagina. As a consequence of this, it guarantees a mild experience until you wish to move on. Being generous with your lady will reward you both with a marvelous enjoyment.

Lying Missionary

Being another desirous sex position, lying missionary is the best to get more fun with the ease of doing since it guarantees enormous satisfaction for both counterparts. The female partner lies straight on her back with the man face-down on top of her, getting full exposure of her body. This position is more desirous due to its simplicity, elegance, comfort, and high level of intimacy. Initial aiming could be a bit difficult for the male, but support from the female counterpart could make it more enjoyable and ensure ease of doing. It gifts both partners an enormous exposure with extreme kissing experience of the bodies and deeper penetration of the penis inside of the vagina, guaranteeing strong stimulation of the clitoris and preventing premature ejaculation. Both partners could malign their bodies deep with face, neck, breasts and chest licking, kissing together with a strong hugging experience. This position provides enthusiastic experience to both partners, by being generous with each other, or wild experience, by being rough with each other.

Folded Missionary

As another subsidiary of the missionary, this position is also quite simple and demanding among the foes due to its higher legitimacy, ease of doing, expressive figure persona and enormous satisfaction for both counterparts. The woman lies down on her back with arms around the back of the man. The only difference is the folded legs of the woman. This allows her to push the hips upward, towards the male partner, to feel and enthusiast deeper vaginal intercourse. Man, being on top, lies face-down on her, going deeper into the vaginal hole till the root of his penis, providing joyous treat of licking and sucking of body parts. For beginners, this is a priority position thanks to its enthusiastic gift of deep penetration, strong and physical vaginal intercourse and intermingling of bodies. This allows kissing and feeling the counterpart with comprehensive outbreaks of hugging. This position delights both partners with unending joy and remembers able sex experience. That is why it drives millions of partners to have sex most of the time in this position.

Tucked Missionary

As a dear relative of folded missionary, tucked type differs in female's legs position, that is bent on the knees, lied towards the abdomen and positioned outside of the male's body. This benefits man by reducing the strain of leaning more and getting tired early. It also encourages man to get more physical and smooth towards the woman by getting frictionless, deeper vaginal penetration, with no barriers across the way, as legs are farther apart. It allows both partners to feel the thorough legitimacy of facial expression reading, hugging tightly, kissing and licking every part of the partner's body, plus a strong inclusion of sex organs. This position allows deeper penetration, with mild experience of frictionless travel and clitoris journey, with favorable experiences for both partners. It allows partners to mingle their bodies with fuller instincts and an extensive experience of kissing and praising the female body as man is on top, lying straight and leaning forward by applying some weight on the female's body. This experience is quite enthusiastic and satisfies both partners.

Wrapped Missionary

This is another most demanding sex position for beginners or efficient partners to get indulge in the mild experience of sex. To get involved in the wrapped position, the woman lies down on her back and wraps her legs around the back of the man, inclusively pressurizing him to stick to her body and feel hot with generous deep penetration. On the other hand, man is kneeling, lying face-down on her with bodies tightly joined, feeling the boobs on his chest and playing with her body by sucking boobs and kissing her face, neck and upper body parts, caressing her hairs and allowing her to hug him tightly and feel the moment with deeper instincts. As you deeply get involved in this position, you will experience an undeniable and unforgettable joy that will last longer and could steer both of you towards sex. The woman also raises her legs and tilts her pelvis, allowing him to smoothly penetrate the vagina, and uses her legs to guide him towards her joy as much as she likes.

Kneeling Missionary

Another desirous position out of the cluster of missionary sex positions is the kneeling missionary. This is closely related to the closed missionary, featuring the male's legs on the outside of women's. This is not as efficient as other missionary positions. As this doesn't allow males to go deep into the vagina and vaginal intercourse, it is quite not efficient enough to fully satisfy the male counterpart. The female partner hugs the male and hangs on her hips to his thighs to feel the deeper intercourse, but doesn't guarantee as always. Being a difficult angle of penetration, this is not the most efficient use of man's length. On the other hand, it benefits the female partner by allowing enormous clitoral stimulation by friction and rubbing of the penis with the inner lips of the vagina, satisfying her with mild joy. This position benefits especially the females who haven't got deeper yet in the vagina.

Woman on Top

This category of positions involves a little dominance of the woman if allowed by the male side. It fills both partners with joys and adventures due to its uniqueness, verities, and enthusiasm. It gives a real sight to the vaginal intercourse, anal gaping and licking or sucking with extreme instinct. No matter in what situation woman remains, being on top of his penis, permits him to pet her breasts, kiss her lips, hug her tightly or hold her buttocks firmly. It also may allow slapping on her ass gently to turn sex into a rough one and increasing the delights with the harsh approach. It is up to the partners to opt either of the two. These positions make her able to control the pace and deepness of entry into her holes and let him observe the female movement with beautiful sights of the penis going in and out of the vagina and anal gap.

Lying Cowgirl

Being a marvelous sex position from the horizon of the woman on top, lying cowgirl is acknowledged by those who give equal voice to their lady. It allows both male and female partners to lie down with the woman face-down on the male partner who is lying on his back. The woman's legs are right above the man's legs and provide less mobility for both partners as man is beneath the woman and less able to deeply penetrate his penis in and out of the vagina. A higher degree of intimacy is guaranteed due to rubbing and extreme intercourse of the penis with the vagina. It also allows both partners to feel and enthusiast sex with unlimited kissing joys and licking adventures. The best pleasure could be gained with the woman positioned a little up from the male's body, allowing him more space to thrust upward with gentle pushes. It gives both partners full exposure with elegant kissing, feeling tightly joined bodies and sucking breasts, guaranteeing marvelous joys and adventures.

Closed Cowgirl

A more joyous sex position with the man lying on his back, straightening his legs, and woman on top with legs closed inside the legs of the male partner. Bodies are bonded tightly with the woman hugging him strongly, providing a sensible and elegant experience with a full vaginal provision and strong clitoris stimulation. Male partner pushes her forward to give deep vaginal intercourse by hands lying on the female's ass. Whereas the female partner encircles her hands around the neck of the male, creating adventures of extreme kissing and licking. This provides a fairly shallow penetration with an edge of easy anal play if partners agree to go inside of the asshole. This position houses the potential to drive both partners crazy and wild by allowing speedy penetration with the sensible feel of vanilla sex. Being crazy in this position will boost sexual pleasures and allow both partners to indulge deep in a sexual intercourse which fairly resists in leaving out even after cumming.

Rodeo

To realize the most depraved desires and enthusiast you, sex is a perfect way out to fulfill the desires that are hovering in your mind for a long time. The man lies on his back, with straight legs and straight body. The woman sits on top of the male partner with her body inclined backward, legs bent in knees and feet stretched out along the body of the male partner. The woman slightly bends her head backward, giving her breasts a full exposure of the air, or slightly bends her face backward, giving her breast's exposure to the male partner. The man puts his hands on the woman's waist or her buttocks while the woman puts her hands backward to support her body, in between the abdomen and arms of the man. This position allows the man to penetrate deeply her holes and give efficient vaginal intercourse as well as deeper anal intercourse since the anal hole is slightly nearer. This will spice up the intercourse, making sex way more exciting and giving a great experience for both male and female partners.

Folded Rodeo

This position is similar to the previous one as the man is lying on his back with straight legs and face towards woman's butt and back. Woman, on the other hand, is on top of the man with back on his side, leaning her face and shoulders forward, hands on his legs to give him relaxation and full room to decide to penetrate deep into her vaginal hole or asshole with painful rubbing and clitoral stimulation. The man could watch every inch of him going inside of the woman, giving him joyous pleasures and unending delights. While, on the other hand, the woman can control the length of the penis going inside her, being able to move forward and backward to adjust her position and let him to go deep or less inside of her. These position enthusiasts both partners with anal joys since anal play is easy in rodeos. Gentle pushes with hands over her buttocks will turn both partners into crazy beasts as the party goes on.

Kneeling Rodeo

Another desirous sex position for those who love cowgirl sex and rodeo positions is kneeling rodeo, as it also enthusiasts the woman by being on top. The man lies on his back with straight body and legs folded on knees in an upward direction. Whereas, the woman sits on his abdomen with penis inclusion and relaxes on his knees by putting her hands. The woman is also on her knees, feet back aligned with his body, giving him full exposure and sight of her back, asshole, vagina and penis inclusion into her holes. This provides the best experience of penis inclusion into the anal mysteries as this enthusiasts both partners with easy access to the anal hole and doubles the joys of the man with sights of every inch going inside her. Whereas, the woman can feel every inch without any resistance and rubbing on the inner lips of the vagina and corners of asshole will make her feel special and satisfied. Gentle pushes could turn both partners into wild beasts due to joys involved.

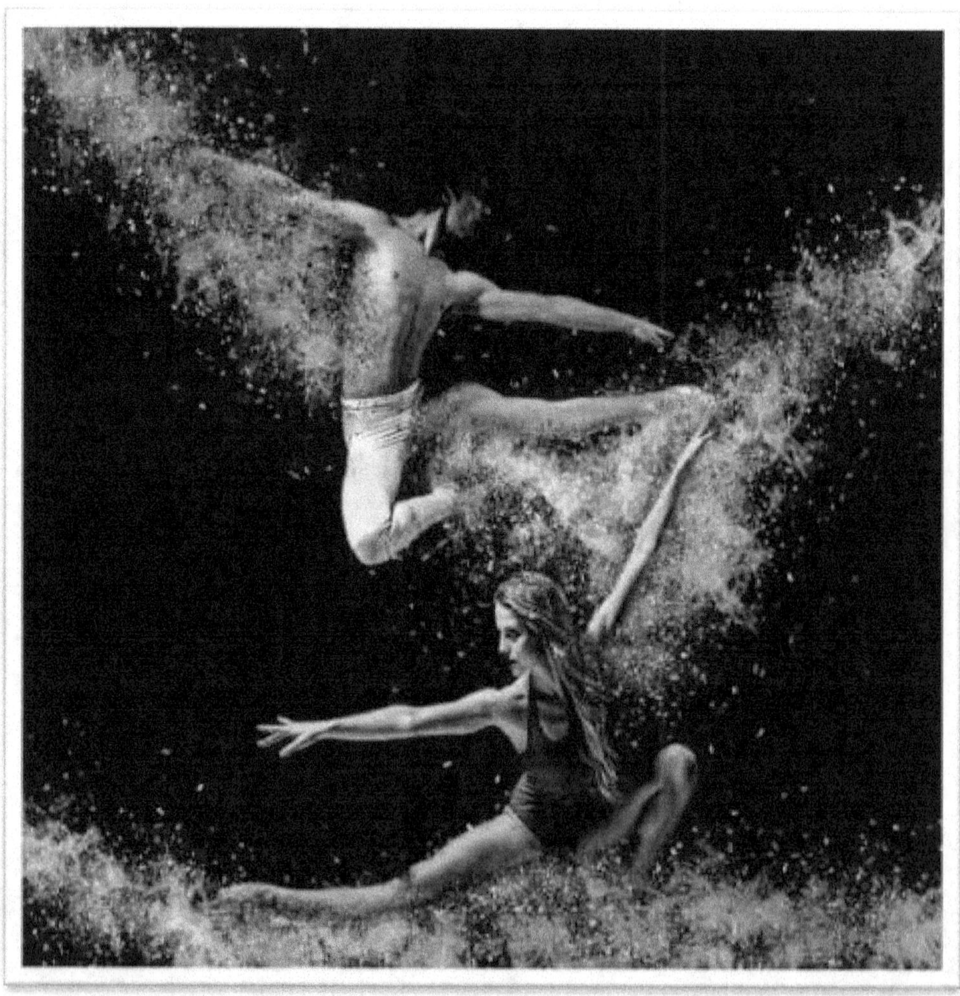

Chapter 8 Advanced positions

- Swing- For this position, the man kneels up, puts his feet on the ground, and reclines on his back. He then lifts his hip only to be supported by the shoulders, the head, and his feet. He may choose to put his hands underneath behind him to act as additional support. The woman stands on top with legs apart the man's knees and then gradually sitting for penetration. This acrobatic location requires a strong back for it tends to be tiresome.

- Wheelbarrow- This position derives its name from the depiction that the couples make as they use it in sex. The man stands upright while the woman stands in front with her hands as support. The man lifts her by the ankles and positions her lips on his sides. The man is left between the woman's legs, making it easy to make a deep penetration and experience a wild and animalistic feeling. It is worth to note that the position requires upper body strength and ability. There is a variation of this position known as the advanced cow, but in this case, the man holds the woman's waist bringing her closer to the groin. This way, the man can control the pace of movement as well as the depth of his thrusts.

- Squeeze- It is a position that makes both partners participate and change roles. The woman lies on her back, facing up and placing her feet on the partner's chest. The position is similar to one formed when you step on the wall while lying on your bed. Chiefly, it puts the man on the wall position facing the woman. Women enjoy this position for it makes them feel relaxed. Men may choose to spice-up this position by rising on their knees, raising the woman's hips off the ground. However, women find this version uncomfortable for it leaves them resting on their upper back. In general, the position is popular for its stimulation of the G-spot.

- Luxurious Lap- The position starts by both partners sitting while facing peachy other. The woman sits between the man's legs and raises her feet to put them on the man's shoulders. Both lean behind placing their hands behind them as support. After the formation, the man draws his partner close to him to find the best angle of insertion. It is a relaxing position for physically fit couples and ensures that they maintain eye contact.

- Web - While it may sound more of a position, the web position is more of a physical feat. It positions the woman in what looks like a mega spider web in a manner that could allow different forms of penetration. The numerous sexually available ways make the man feel free to work; however, he finds fit. The artistic nature of the web makes it easy to create a different sexual position. However, the web may be costly or require extensive maintenance.

- Crab- As an advanced sex position, you must be sure that this one too requires physical fitness, especially on your hands. The man starts by lying while facing upwards and raising himself to support by hands and feet. The woman then sits on him and lies on his lap and stretching her hands out to reach the ground for support. If she is tall enough, her feet may reach the ground under the man's butt. She then lowers onto the penis and raises her pelvis. Through teamwork, you should get a real workout.

- Ladder- In this position, the woman hangs on the man who comes from behind. The position requires a degree of maneuvers. The man stands behind the woman holding her hands towards him. The woman then steps just above the man's knees as he bends to make her feel comfortable. They then adjust their bodies to allow for a smooth slip. Notably, couples engaging in this position should be sure of their stamina and keeping of balance.

- Arc Love- The position requires that the man sits on a flat platform extending the feet in front of him. The woman should then crawl up to him on her knees and start straddling him. She should make herself comfortable and arch into a back end while lowering into the erect penis. Proper caution should be taken to avoid straining the lower back too much. The woman could also rest her head between his feet and grab his ankles. At this time, the man should lean forward and start the action.

- Propeller- As the name suggests, this position requires one partner to act as a propeller. The man starts by lying on top of the woman in the traditional missionary form. After complete penetration, the partner then starts rotating around like a propeller as the woman supports and guides him in the spin. The position requires partners to have sheer coordination to avoid hitting each other's head or similar incidents. The woman should be sure to lift the feet as they pass over her head as the man is busy screwing things up.

- X-shaped- It is a position that required a degree of control and coordination. The man should lie face up while the woman straddles on him as she turns around. The woman's back should be pointed towards him and should lower herself to position well on the penis. Her legs should be extended towards the man' shoulders while relaxing her torso between his feet. After ultimately forming the x-shape, the woman should then slide up and down and utilize his feet for enhanced thrusting.

- Head Squeeze- It is one of the games considered as not suitable for the faint-hearted. It is a challenging one and starts by lying flat and face up. As a woman, you should use your hands to support the back while making a perpendicular inclination while feet lifted high. The man should kneel and grab your hips up as he brings his knees close to your shoulders. The position allows you to be steady as you expose the most critical area of the moment. By holding on to his thighs, you can adjust and leverage your pace and position.
- Booty- The position provides a challenge of gaining momentum but provides a smooth sexy ride once mass. The man sits stretching his feet in front of him. The posture allows the woman to face downwards and lies between the partner's feet, pulling her feet behind the man. She then lowers herself to access the erect penis. The position is excellent for its association with freedom and

ability to engage the hands for killer workouts and biceps.

- Vixen- Depending on your flexibility, you could use this position to go a long way. It provides a deep penetration making it worth trying. The man should stand upright in front of the receiver. The woman puts her hands around his neck and his arms around her lower back. He then helps her prop her two feet on his shoulders. The man may opt to make a knee bend to make a full-on jaw-dropper on this move.

- Stairs- The position brings a new meaning to sex and romance. The woman kneels on an elevated platform such as a staircase while the man kneels on the lowercase. Both face the stairs while the woman's behind locks with the man's groin. The man holds her hips to penetrate her from behind as she reaches up to stairs or the banister.

- Profound Impact- The fact that the position requires the woman to prop her legs makes it most preferred for men who like going as deep as they can. The woman gets on her side and lifts one of her legs while the man straddles the other. The man should kneel and make her discover the hidden spots in her. On trying this position, you will enjoy not only the relaxation but also the easy access to the clitoris.

- The extensive list proves that sexual positions could be varied to offer new and more refreshing outcomes. A relentless mind and a go-getter mentality would be critical in attempting these techniques. Nevertheless, numerous trials and practice are a sure course to perfection.

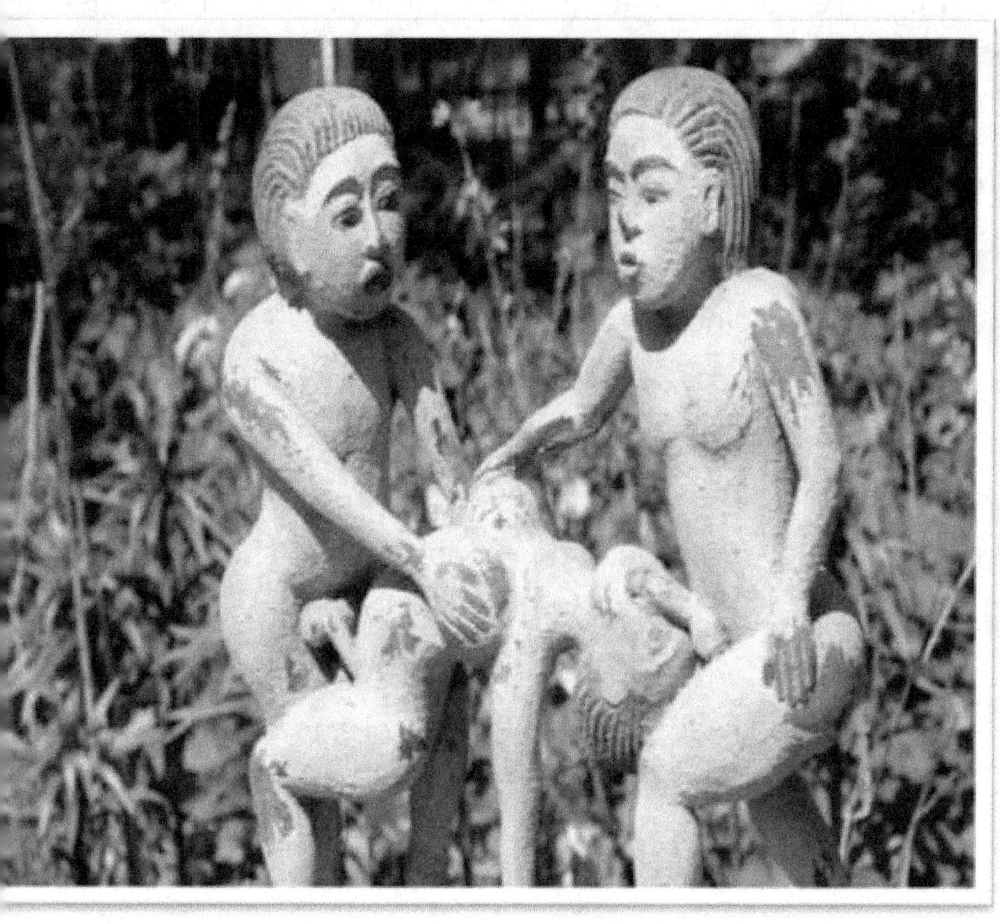

Chapter 9 The Kama Sutra Techniques Related To Kissing

The mouth is one of the most sensitive parts of a human's body. It can give you pleasurable sensations and help you achieve a heightened urge for intense lovemaking. This body part is also versatile–you may use your tongue and lips to lick, suck, kiss, nibble, or nuzzle any part of your lover's body.

Actually, kissing is considered as an art. The Kama Sutra appreciates its potential in expressing passion and affection. The book shows this appreciation by explaining different kinds of kisses and when each kind of kiss must be used. Regardless of their intensity, kisses on the lips combine three senses: smell, taste, and touch. As you probably know, these senses can create powerful physical and emotional responses.

There are different kinds of kisses available, ranging from slight touches to deep penetrations (i.e. using the tongue). This chapter will describe each type of kiss in detail:

1. <u>Turned</u> –This kiss occurs when one of the lovers turns up his/her partner's face by holding the chin and kissing.

Note: This kind of kiss evokes gentleness from the couple. Use it to start the foreplay or while making love (i.e. in a face-to-face standing or sitting position).

2. <u>Bent</u>–Here, the man must bend his head toward that of his partner. The woman must do the same. The lovers must hold this position while kissing.

Note: When using this technique, make sure that your head is slightly angled to one side. This head position allows you to achieve total lip contact and tongue penetration. Many people use this technique as their main weapon during foreplay.

3. <u>Pressed</u>–This kiss has two versions:

4. When you are pressing your partner's lower lip forcibly

5. When you hold your partner's lower lip, touch it with your tongue, and kiss it forcibly.

Note:Many people don't consider this as an actual kiss. It's more of a passionate introduction to kissing.

6. <u>Straight</u>–This kind of kiss occurs when the lips of a man touches that of his partner. Here, the lovers'heads must be straight (i.e. not bent or turned).

Note:With this type of kiss, tongue penetration is extremely difficult. For this reason, you can't use the straight kiss to express passion. You must perform a straight kiss to show affection and desire.

7. <u>The Upper Lip Kiss</u> –This kiss occurs when the man kisses his partner's upper lip. The woman, in turn, kisses the man's lower lip.

8. <u>Clasping</u>–In this kiss, one of the lovers must take the lips of his/her partner between his/her own. However, women only accept this kind of kiss if their partner has no mustache (for obvious reasons).

Note:This move is now called"French Kiss." This kind of kiss requires excellent oral hygiene (again, for obvious reasons).

9. <u>The Kisses of a Young Girl</u> –According to the Kama Sutra, the couple must perform

kissing moderately if it's their first time to make love.

10.   Throbbing –Here, the girl touches her partner's lips as they kiss. Then, she must move her lower lip while keeping the upper one stationary.

11.   Nominal–In this kiss, the girl simply uses her lips to touch that of her partner.

12.   Touching –With this technique, the girl uses her tongue to touch her partner's lips. Meanwhile, she should close her eyes and hold the hands of her partner.

13.   <u>The Kiss That Can Trigger Passion</u> –This kiss helps a woman to arouse her lover if he is sleeping. Here, the woman must look at her lover's face, kiss him passionately, and show her sexual desires.

Note: As this technique shows, women must feel comfortable initiating passionate activities.

14.   <u>The Kiss That Can Wake a Person Up</u> –This is a variation of the kiss described above. With this technique, the man kisses his partner and expresses his desire to make love. This kiss is particularly effective when the man comes home late at night and finds his partner sleeping.

Kissing Your Partner's Body

It is true that the lips and breasts are sensitive to kisses. However, almost all body parts (e.g. limbs) can produce pleasurable sensations when kissed. Generally, body parts that are close to a person's genitals are sensitive to touches of the tongue and lips. This section of the book will explain the different techniques that you can use in kissing your partner's body.

For the Breasts –Men should apply light kisses on the entire breasts and suck (or nibble) the nipples gently. Since most women find nipple stimulation extremely arousing, men must pay special attention to their partner's nipples.

Important Note: Male lovers must spend sufficient time on fondling and kissing their partner's breasts. This is because most women find breast massages physically satisfying and emotionally exciting. Actually, some women feel dissatisfied if their partner ignores their breasts in favor of their vagina.

For the Thighs –When kissed, the thighs produce pleasing, erotic sensations. These sensations run throughout your partner's body, increasing his/her sexual desires.

<u>For the Back</u> –The Kama Sutra says that you should lick or kiss your partner's spine lightly. This action will send powerful sensations to his/her entire body (i.e. from his/head down to his/her toes).

Licking And Kissing

You must pay attention to sexually sensitive areas such as nipples and breasts. You will get more enjoyment from penetration the longer you delay it. If you can stimulate your body and that of your partner to the fullest through kissing and licking, you'll get more rewards from penile penetration once it occurs.

According to the Kama Sutra, a great way to boost your partner's anticipation is by kissing his/her body systematically and/or giving him/her a"tonguebath."Tongue bathing is a technique in which a lover uses his/her tongue to explore his/her partner's body.

Important Tips About Kissing

This section of the book will give you excellent tips that can improve your kisses.

- You can boost the stimulating effect of your kiss by combining it with gentle strokes of your fingers.
- Kissing your partner's body isn't enough. You have to supplement this with sensual strokes and touches.
- Kiss your partner's neck, back, ears, lips, and cheeks.
- You can perform most of the kisses discussed above while standing or sitting with your partner.
- To make your kisses more sensual, kiss your partner's lower and upper lips in turn.

How To Bite Sensually

In ancient India, biting was a crucial aspect of sexual stimulation. This is the reason why the Kama Sutra describes different biting techniques. In general, you can bite almost any part of your partner's body. Also, bites can take the form of playful nipping (for teasing your partner), prolonged sucking (which leaves a noticeable mark), or forceful gripping (using the lover's teeth).

This chapter will explain the different Kama Sutra Techniques related to biting.

- <u>The Boar's Bite</u> –The Kama Sutra recommends this bite for people who want to mark their partner's shoulder. This bite involves multiple rows of marks separated by reddish gaps. Some individuals also use this technique to mark the breasts of their partners. In general, people who are sexually intense use this technique during lovemaking.

Important Note: Recent researches have shown that females appreciate biting while making love to their partners. Males, however, are often ambivalent about being bitten or biting their lovers. Psychologists say that since men have larger muscles than women, they prefer to show their passion through body movements than through their teeth.

- <u>Broken Cloud</u> –This biting technique involves a circle of unequal marks. The inequality of the bite marks results from the spaces between a person's teeth. According to the Kama Sutra, this technique is excellent for leaving bite marks on a woman's breasts.

- **<u>Different Love Bites</u>** –The following list shows the biting techniques that you can use while making love to your partner:

  - Point –You can accomplish this technique by biting your partner's skin using your two front teeth.

  - Hidden –This technique leaves a noticeable redness on the skin you bit. However, there should be no other visible marks.

  - Line of Points –In this biting technique, you will bite a small area of the skin using most of your teeth.

  - Coral and Jewels –You must use your lips and teeth when doing this biting technique. Your lips serve as the coral and your teeth serve as the jewels.

  - Line of Jewels –This technique occurs when you bite you partner using all of your teeth.

  - Swollen –Here, you must use your teeth to press down your partner's skin.

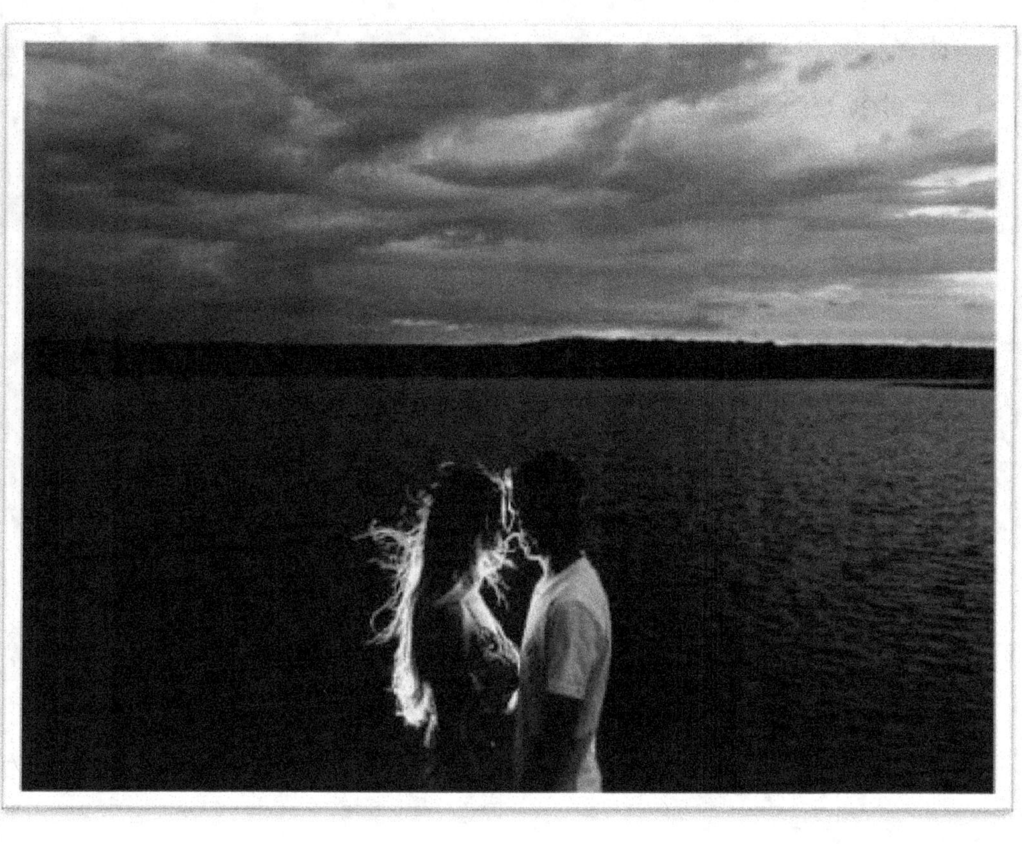

Chapter 10 Tantric Sex Positions

Accepted to go back nearly a large number of years, Tantric sex is an old Eastern otherworldly practice. Like yoga or Zen, its motivation is illumination—and the way of thinking rises above the room into all parts of life. In the Tantric view, sex and orgasm equals profound mindfulness at its pinnacle. Furthermore, when Shiva (male vitality) and Shakti (female vitality) participate in one sexual association, it is accepted to be the most elevated purpose of illumination.

Best of all, we all hold the way to Tantric sex: breath. If you can keep your body loose and your mind clear of the unremarkable, your "inward goddess" can be completely present. Utilizing your breath can spread orgasmic vitality from your private parts through your whole body. This all-over shivering, thus, prompts an increasingly personal association with your accomplice.

Also, notwithstanding all the discussion of an unreasonably useful for-words orgasm, the huge "O" is not the objective of Tantra. Rather, it is progressively about being at the time and riding a rush of sensation and excitement (yours and your partner's). If you center around getting to one huge explosion toward the end, you may pass up huge amounts of other "orgasmic delights" occurring in your bodies en route. Tantric educators guarantee that notwithstanding more full orgasms, ladies experience them all the more rapidly since they figure out how to turn out to be increasingly loose and sharpened.

1. Make a sacrosanct space.

Change your room. Stir your faculties with blossoms, fragrant healing oils, scented candles, new organic products, and chocolates. Incorporate exotic textures like silk for included tangible components—regardless of whether it is your sheets or your unmentionables.

2. Shake your body alive.

You've opened up every one of these spots where there is pressure and expanded the affectability, permitting joy in. If you have intercourse subsequent to doing that, almost certainly, you will have an entire body orgasm."

3. Inhale and shake.

Sit on the bed or floor, confronting your accomplice (you are on his lap). Start by shutting your eyes, and utilize your creative mind to watch your breath move all through your body. Begin to enable your breath to go three crawls underneath your stomach catch. Start shaking like you are in a recliner, pushing your chest ahead as you breathe in, and shaking back as you breathe out.

The astonishing association that you will feel will take your breath away. Your vitality fields get together, so you are both in a similar state and are significantly more touchy to one another. It is exceptionally electric.

4. Offer a Tantric kiss.

Keep on sitting on his lap and shake together—you breathing in while he's breathing out and the other way around. As you breathe out, be cognizant that you are offering all of yourself to your accomplice. At that point kiss and offer the breath. Intercourse is not even important in light of the fact that you are so consolidated. Tantra is tied in with jumping profoundly into want and joy. If you feel better and delighted, at that point you are in good shape.

Tantric sex is not about system, it is not about positions. It is absolutely not about the extreme flexibility you in some cases find in books! So what are tantric sex positions? For what reason do they make a difference? Which positions would it be a good idea for you to know? Tantric sex happens when two typified human spirits meet up in absolute nearness and receptiveness and through the bliss of their sexual association stir to association with the Divine. It is an unconstrained, streaming and articulate radical articulation of affection and closeness at the most profound level.

Be that as it may, tantric sex is additionally a craftsmanship, a deliberately imaginative weaving of structure. The Taoist custom (firmly identified with Tantra) talks about sexual "gongfu" or sexual authority. Dominance of any work of art calls for ability and method. A couple's voyage into tantric sex will be significantly helped by sharing a bed of hues, both striking and unobtrusive, to paint their perfect work of art. Having the option to appreciate the play of positions during lovemaking is a piece of that bed. Tantric sex is apt sex.

Tantric sex is about profound amazing quality however it is additionally about enthusiastic change and this is the place positions are significant. The situating of a few's bodies in connection to one another and to the enthusiastic fields of the earth and the universe can make the incredible vibrational resonances, arrangements or polarities that are the vigorous establishment of otherworldly association.

The Taoists especially got this. In old China, sex "specialists" would recommend specific love making positions to adjust the body's qi and recuperate disease.

The establishment of the human vitality framework is the Central Channel which goes through the center of the body from the private parts to the head. Along the Central Channel vitality focuses or Chakras capacity to encapsulate specific human possibilities.

The positions utilized in tantric love making help to open and adjust these focuses to the point where our full Divine potential is typified.

For every one of the tantric love making positions I will portray, I'll clarify precisely how they influence the Central Channel and chakras.

The positions depicted are not fascinating or obscure. They will presumably as of now be a piece of the collection of most cherishing couples. They do not require accomplishments of readiness or astonishing quality and adaptability. Essentially they typify and express profound, delicate closeness. They offer you a strong establishment for the enthusiastic work inside tantra. They are a beginning stage from which a couple can investigate the spirit move of tantric lovemaking.

These sex positions are in no way, shape or form the main ones proper to tantra. A bold and innovative couple will find a huge number of conceivable outcomes and varieties. A few positions will suit a few couples superior to other people. Body shape and size, by and large and private, will have a direction here. What's more, kindly do not feel you need to work however the lovemaking positions as an everyday practice. Give them a chance to emerge unexpectedly from the progression of your affection play.

The estimation of these positions is not constrained to penetrative sex. These positions are beautiful ways basically to snuggle and be close. You can likewise utilize them for tantric massage.

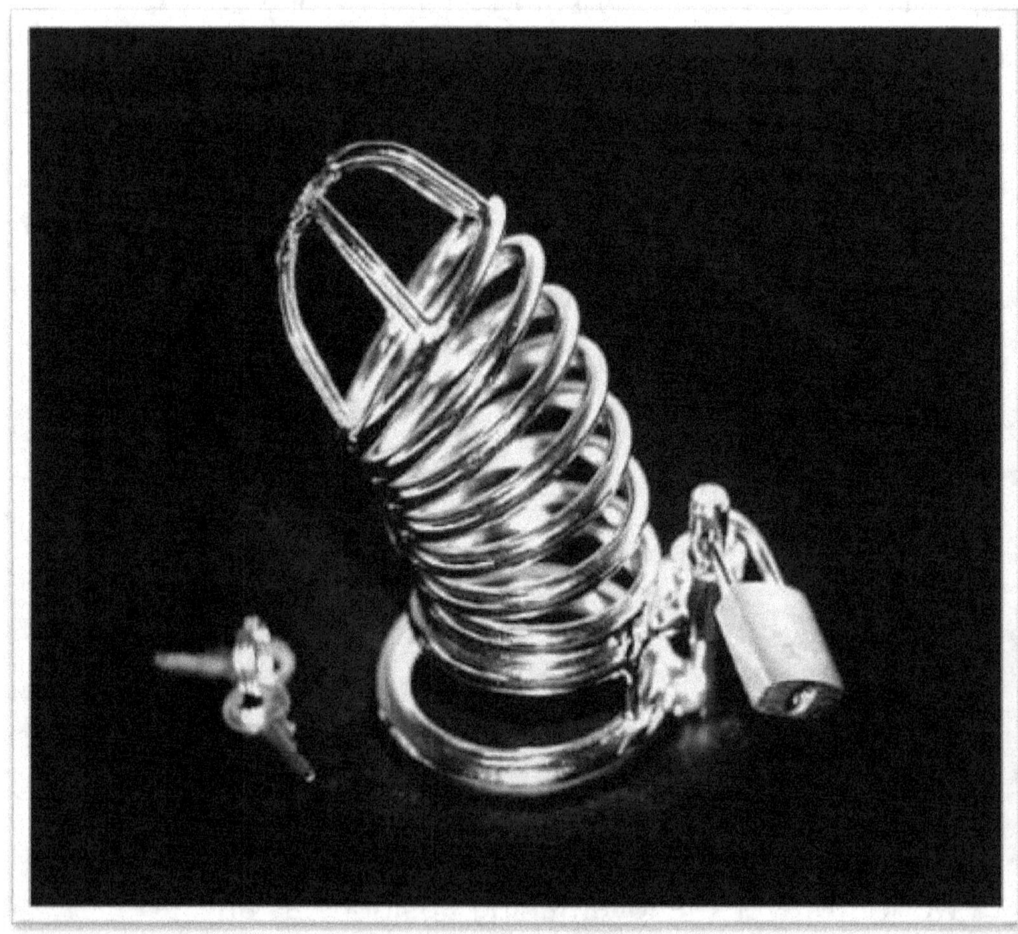

Chapter 11 Sex Variants

Sex Toys

Sex toys are devices or object a person may use to cause sexual stimulation. The tools are made to replace the pleasure that human genitalia would provide. Although there are vibrating toys, other forms of toys may provide pleasure without having to vibrate. These toys are readily available in sex shops and are available in a variety of types and purposes. It would be advisable for you to incorporate sex toys if only your partner advocates for it. You could use them before, during, and after sexual intercourse to initiate, maintain, and prolong sexual stimulation. This chapter will provide a broad perspective about the type, usage, and limitations of sex toys

Types of Sex Toys

- *Electro stimulators*- These toys are available for both men and women and use electricity for stimulation. They work when placed on nerve endings, where they send signals to the brain. As a result, the brain releases pleasure hormones which then may lead to orgasm.

- *Penetrative Toys*- These are sex toys that are meant to make a penetration for sexual pleasure. They include a dildo which is a vibrating object used to penetrate either the anus or the vagina. Although there are different shapes of dildos, most resembles the shape of the penis. The most common types of dildos include strap-on and double penetration. Similarly, a horseshoe toy penetrates both the vagina and the anus at the same time to provide maximum stimulation and pleasure. A sex machine combines penetration with a rotational movement while a kegel exerciser improves the muscle tone of the vagina. There are love balls commonly inserted and lodged in the vagina for prolonged stimulation and eventually orgasm. Anal beads work similarly with the butt plugs, which are also embedded in the anus and make a smooth rotation to cause stimulation. Men like a massage on the prostate and enhance orgasm. Glass sex toys are made of clear glass and may sometimes aid in medical purposes. The glasses act as perfect temperature regulators as they penetrate in the anus or the vagina. Vibrators offer most of their stimulation through vibrating and come in different shapes and sizes. Some of them are customized on the client's preference, making them diverse and multipurpose. Anal vibrators are meant for anal insertion while bullet ones are inserted in the vagina and may incorporate a finger or a cock ring. The curved G-spot vibrators are curved to access the woman's G-spot.

- *Nipple Toys-* These are toys meant to stimulate the nipples through their sensitive material and shape. Some may need a varying degree of pressure to be effective while others, such as suction devices, use glass or rubber. They apply to a woman or a man with the use of other toys in other body parts.
- *Penile Toys-* These toys are meant to cause stimulation to the penis. For example, the pocket pussies or the artificial vaginas are tubes made of soft tissues to make it feel

like a real vagina. A variation of the device may incorporate a system similar to that of a milking machine. A cock harness is used to maintain erection and is worn around the penis. Similarly, cock rings are used to hold the blood in the penis to maintain an erection and may have a clitoris stimulator to perform its duty during sex. The cock rings may also vibrate to ensure that both partners get the best from the toy. A sleeve is a cylindrical device that is open on both ends and could be used to form mutual masturbation. There is also a penis extension that is hollow and shorter than a dildo. They are worn on the tip of the penis to achieve deep penetration. It is advisable to wear a condom to hold the toy from falling off.

Factors to Consider When Selecting Sex Toys

Sex toys are becoming popular, especially among the youth and couples. While there are different types of sex toys, some could be exciting and others intimidating. It would be very tricky trying out a toy that you have never used before. For that reason, you should make the following considerations to get the best toy for you and maximize enjoyment and pleasure.

1. Start easy- When selecting your first sex toy, you should start with the simplest toys there is. This way, you can work up to more advanced toys in the future. Start steadily to avoid disappointments and intimidations.
2. Cleanliness- It is essential to keep your body clean and hygienic, especially your genitals. Therefore, ensure you select sex toys that are cleaned easily and less likely to attract bacteria while in storage.
3. Preference- It is common to find that what works for the service provider is not what will work for you. For that reason, you should ensure you acquire a sex toy depending on your likes and preference.
4. Research- Finding reviewed products online has become simpler; hence, the importance of understanding a sex toy before purchasing or trying it.
5. Storage- Extra care is needed when storing sex toys. They could react to materials

placed near them. It is common to find silicone or latex toys looking melted.

6. Consult with your partner- It is for your good to be upfront, open, and honest to your partner about the desires you have with sex toys. Similarly, let them know your preference and use their reaction to judge whether they are okay with it.

7. Maintain Communication- It is the most crucial part of sex, especially when using sex toys. This way, your partner lets you know the part that is stimulated by the toy making it possible to discover additional erogenous zones.

8. Maintain Safety- It is advisable to use these toys for the sole purpose for which they are meant. You should be cautious when using these toys for good sex. Notably, problems occur whenever users fail to follow instructions.

Various Uses of Sex Toys

- *Normalize Sensitivity-* Partner may have difficulties having intercourse due to their bodies being hypersensitive. It is a common scenario among new couples. Their genitals may not be exposed to sex before and require preparations for the real act. Sex toys could be used slightly to stimulate the genitals, and they will be ready to have sex with time.

- *Foreplay-* Sex toys are best in causing stimulations, especially for couples, for they are multipurpose and continuous. Partners could use the different types of toys to stimulate each other before they engage in actual sex. It would work miracles for less physically fit couples. It also saves time that partners could take to achieve stimulation.

- *Maintain Stimulation-* Sex toys do not disappoint when incorporated in sex. They may be used to cause stimulation to both partners making sex more pleasurable. When using sex positions that have limited caressing and kissing, sex toys could be the ultimate solution.

- *Prolong Stimulation-* In this case, the partners wish to prolong the stimulation even after orgasm and sex. As they relax after sex, couples could continue using the toys to make the stimulation last longer. It could work for men with erectile dysfunction for it aids in a prolonged erection.

- *Third Partner-* Sex toys could be used in case one of the partners has passed out or cannot reach certain sensitive areas. For instance, a partner would prefer concurrent stimulation on both the anus and the vagina. The sex toys would take one responsibility as the partner handles the other.

With all these uses, you are sure to find the best sex toy that will work for you and your partner. There are few evitable cons of sex toys while the pros make them a must use.

Pros of Sex Toys

1. *Enhances Body Knowledge-* The use of sex toys during sex helps partners explore each other bodies and understand the part with more sensory stimulation.
2. *Enhances Sexual Pleasure-* The combination of these toys with sex provides additional pleasure.
3. *Self Confidence-* While using sex toys, you are sure that sexual stimulation is

guaranteed making you aim at attaining satisfaction.

4. *Quick Orgasm-* The hyper intensive stimulation caused by sex toys reduces the time a partner would require to attain an orgasm. For that reason, sex starts at the right time with little effort applied.

5. *Control Sexual Needs-* Sex toys could be used by either partner for sexual stimulation.

6. *Fosters Love-* The exploration of your partner's genitals as well as communication as you try out sex toys removes barriers and enhances mutual connections.

7. *Prevents STIs-* The use of sex toys means that genitals may not need to make contact thus preventing the spread of sexually transmitted Infections.

8. *Improves Performance-* The sensitivity associated with sex toys boosts the partner's morale, making them perform above par.

9. *Prevents Unwanted Pregnancy-* The fact that sex toys do not ejaculate makes it safe for the woman from impregnation.

Cons

1. *Toxicity*- Materials used to make sex toys may be toxic to your body although few severe cases have come up.
2. *Infections*- Untidy and contaminated devices may carry bacteria that may end up infecting your body. For that reason, you should ensure that your sex toys are kept safely in a clean environment.

Oral Sex

This form of sex involves the use of the mouth to stimulate the external reproductive organs of your partner. It goes well when combined with sucking, nibbling, blowing, and licking. *Fellatio* is when a man is receiving oral sex, and *cunnilingus* is oral sex on a woman. In fellatio, the giver of oral sex uses the mouth to stimulate the penis and the scrotum of the man.

On the other hand, cunnilingus involves using the mouth to stimulate the clitoris, vulva, and the openings of the vagina. Besides, oral sex done on the anus is called *analingus.* It is worth noting that using the mouth to stimulate other body parts such as the lips and breasts is not oral sex. Nevertheless, oral sex is an enjoyable and intimate practice for sexy couples. There has been so much misinformation and mystery surrounding this form of sex that it is amazingly punishable in some jurisdictions. For that reason, you should understand oral sex and decide on whether to make it part of a romantic relationship.

Anal Sex

It is a form of sex where the penetration occurs at the anus. The practice happens intending to cause sexual stimulation and play. Therefore, it does not have to end in penetration necessarily. The play may involve stimulating the rectum, bum, or the anus. Note that this form of sex should not be a goal for you to achieve but a pleasure that you choose. Tickling or massaging the outer part of the butt hole is also considered as anal sex for it offers stimulation and delight just as other forms of sex. There are various ways you could stimulate your partner through the anus, and it can be concurrent for both of you. By mastering the following common anal sex positions, you gain additional knowledge on how to get down on your partner.

Anal Sex Positions

- *Missionary-* This position mostly involves deep penetration as the man is on top of the woman. The position offers double stimulation if the woman is male. There are numerous variations of this technique, and the man remains in control of pace, rhythm, and depth of penetration. The woman could raise the hip to enhance position the partners face the same direction while lying on a flat platform. The man enters from behind, forming a spoon shape. In this case, the woman remains in full control of the intercourse. This position offers added stimulation as hands are free to caress and a maintained complete body contact.
- *Doggy-* It can be performed with both partners kneeling or standing. The woman may bend to expose the anus for the man who stands erect behind. It offers a clear view of the penetration and reduces obstruction from the rest of the body. The partners may support each other to avoid

falling off. The man may hold the woman's waist as the holds ion a chair.

- *Receiver on Top- as* the name states, this position has the woman on top of the man. It leaves more control to the woman who decides what pace, speed, and depth to achieve. The man lies on a flat platform, and the only effort he could apply is raising the hips to penetrate deeper or make thrusts. They may decide to take different variations which may diversify the level of stimulation.

- *Posture seven-* It is a position you are likely to find in manuals depicting the posture made in sex from behind. The woman lies on a flat platform allowing the man straddles the lower legand lift it to his elbow or shoulders. This position makes the partners make a posture similar to number seven. Although most couples find this position as acrobatic, others perceive it as comfortable, especially if they have health problems or concerns.

Best Practices for Safe Anal Sex

There are various ways in which you could explore anal sex. The variance makes couples curious about positions and penetration. If you are ready to find out ways to explore anal play safely and pleasurably, you should exercise these steps.

- *Research*- If you are reading this point, you are on the right track of perfecting in anal sex. It is advisable to understand the organs involved to make the right decisions and moves. Specifically, you should understand the pressure- the reaction of your anus as well as that of your partner. You should also understand the occurrence of stimulation occurs after the application of pressure on the ventral walls of the anus
- *Take Easy*- If you are new to anal play and sex, you should take it slow and avoid rushing for orgasm. Time is of the essence as you explore the prostate gland, anal canal, and the sphincter muscles. You should help each other understand what works and what fails. If you feel overwhelmed by negative and stressful emotions, you should

relax and breathe out. Notably, the pain might be a sign that something is wrong.

- *Communicate-* Your partner should be ready to try out the new technique before you bump on them for a quickie. It includes opening your mind, and communicating your feelings and suggestions, trying the unique experience. If they are in for it, ensure you combine it with caressing, and other fantasy for it does not only involve penetration.
- *Be Safe-* Anal sex is not a rush thing and requires proper preparations before penetration. The anus requires caution as you insert relatively larger objects. It is advisable to start with your finger as you gradually adjust sizes and observing the reaction. Ensure that the objects you put in the anus have a flared base to prevent them from being sucked into the rectum. Chiefly, most beginners incorporate effective lube to make it safe and comfortable.
- *Cleanliness-* The taboo aspect of anal sex makes it more arousing for couples. For that reason, they believe that sex must be dirty to be considered effective. However, if you

are engaged in anal sex, some aspects will need extra care. Direct contact of the anal fluids and the vagina may transfer bacteria that inhabit the anus. You could use a latex condom to avoid this direct contact or wash thoroughly before penetration.

Pros of Anal Sex

- *Immunity-* In general sex offers fantastic health benefits. Specifically, anal sex boosts your immune system for it aids in blood circulation as you are involved in sexual exercises. The physical fitness makes you remain in good shape and introduce antibodies that fight off other conditions.
- *Appeal-* Anal sex offers a stimulating appeal on men's prostate as well as the vagina. The nerve endings in these areas are more likely to come into contact with the groin of the man. Consequently, the sensitivity makes the partner experience the appeal and enjoy the intercourse.
- *Nerve Ending-* This form of sex seeks to explore the nerve endings found in the anus. The partners can compare the sensitivity as

well as the degree of stimulation possible. This way, the partners can decide on making various forms of sex, depending on their preference.

- *Clearing-* The penetration of a penis or any other object in the anus is likely to clear the way out for excretion as a form of sex, anal sex aids in bowel movement keeping the woman healthy. Rubbing of the anus increases the blood flow enhances standard blood pressure and digestion.

- *Pleasure-* The fact that reproduction is rare in anal sex makes it solely for fun. Men enjoy sex for the find the anus as tighter as compared to other openings such as the vaginal or the mouth. It also makes them feel dominant and rebellious a sense that feeds their instincts. Women enjoy anal sex due to the sensitivity of the nerve endings around the anus. They also experience stimulation in their clitoris if men use missionary position for anal sex.

- *Intimacy-* Before anal sex happens; the partner must have had mutual trust and transparency. Partners have nerve, insecurity, and privacy issues when it comes to giving in for anal sex. This form of sex requires partners to put aside their reputation and physical requirements. The men treat it as an unusual step by the woman to please him. The women take it as a man's way to show that they are ready to explore them.

- *Contraceptive-* Practicing means that you have no plans to get kids. Similarly, you may use this form of sex when your partner senses that she may get pregnant. It is meant to put out the tension among women reliving them for a great and pleasurable session ahead.

- *Beneficial Semen-* exposure to semen reduces the chances of contracting breast cancer and nausea, and the same case applies in anal sex. When the fluid comes into contact with the woman's body, they are likely to cause increased energy, reduces stress, increased libido, and mental alertness.

- *Diversity-* Anal sex has incorporated different aspects that are interesting to people who felt bored with sex. Partners find this form of sex as a way to introduce something new in their relationship and sex life. It is the best solution for long term relationships partners who would like to make things fun.

- *Timelessness-* Unlike vaginal sex, anal sex can be done anytime without having to wait for days when the woman has a period. Sex is made convenient, and the partner does not need to wait for days to have sexual satisfaction.

Cons

- *Tearing-* Hard thrusts in the anus could cause skin fractures of the rectum. It affects the soft tissues making up the anus. These tears could develop into sores and lead to a severe health condition.
- *HPV-* You might be infected with HPV as you engage in anal sex. The virus may lead to cancer of the anus.
- *HIV-* Although anal sex prevents pregnancy, it does not on the side of STIs. If you fail to

use protection, you may pass or contract HIV from your partner.

- *Prolapsed Anus*- Although it is a rare occurrence, practicing hardcore sex may be hazardous for you or your partner.
- *Poop*- Anal sex is associated with coming into contact with fecal matter. However, this should not come as a surprise, and you should learn how to deal with the issue sexually.

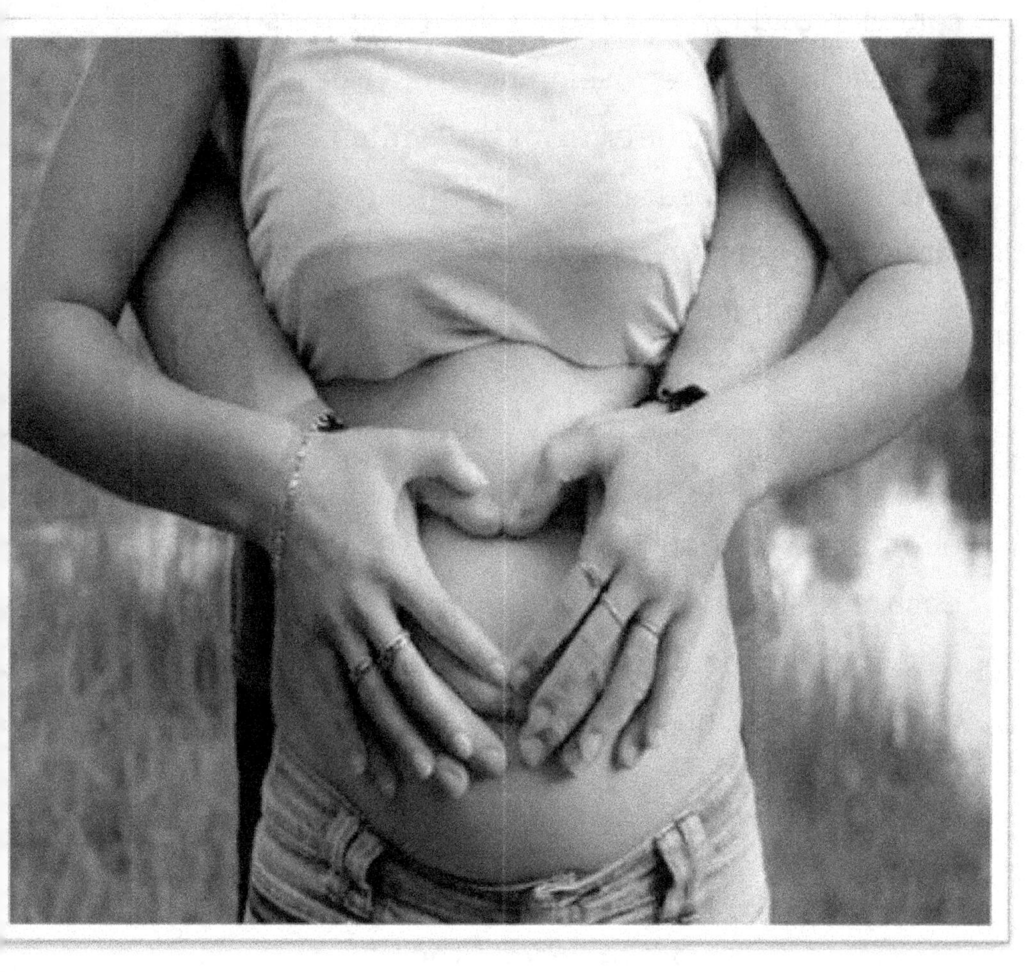

Chapter 12 Sex in Pregnancy

Pregnancy is the ultimate result for couples who had 1 sessions may have been a result of the urge to conceive and make a family. Most partners lose interest in sex after designing or if their partners conceive. If you suffer from the same condition, you should take measures to ensure that you do not lose interest in intimacy due to a short term condition. You may have difficulties expressing your feelings for each other due to concerns over pregnancy. It is safe to have sex during pregnancy and may be beneficial for you and the unborn. It is worth noting that there is a need to be cautious when having sex in at this time to ensure that you do not cause trouble. For that reason, you should make the following considerations for a safe and intimate session during pregnancy.

Considerations for Sex in Pregnancy

- Discuss: It is an essential aspect of sex during pregnancy as the partners should be comfortable and relaxed for an intimate session. The discussion should involve the positions that you will incorporate throughout the session as well as the pace and depth of penetration. Besides, you should get a doctor's approval after doing the necessary check-ups that will give the go-ahead or make reservations.

- Limitations: You should also understand the barriers that are associated with sex during pregnancy. They include keeping a low paced performance and making the session as intimate and straightforward as possible. Besides, other limitations should be observed to ensure that you do not affect the pregnancy and specifically the unborn baby. It includes avoiding combining anal sex and vaginal sex as it may lead to the transfer of bacteria.
- Records: While having sex during pregnancy, you should ensure that it does not bring complication to the woman or the unborn baby. Avoid engaging in this form of sex if your partner has a history of miscarriage.
- History: You must have known your partner if she is pregnant for you. For that reason, you should ensure that the activity does not

affect the timing of her labor. Similarly, you should look out for the history of membrane eruption that is mostly associated with deep penetration and hard-hitting. Membrane eruption is as a result of leakages of the amniotic fluid that acts as a protector from external factors.

- Cervix: You need to take your partner for a thorough check-up of the cervix to ensure that it is in the perfect condition that makes it right for sex. Ignoring this consideration may lead to other severe conditions that would require special attention from medical experts.
- Positions: The big bump in pregnancy may act as a facilitator or an obstruction during sex. Therefore, you should opt for flexible positions that make it easy for both of you. The side by side rear entry position acts as a perfect example of positions that would be easy and sexually stimulating.
- Make Necessary Reports: You should check on your partner every time you have sex to ensure that there are no abnormalities or straining. Make appropriate reports to the

doctor if you detect problems such as pain or discharge during sex. These discharges may include blood which is a clear indication of a severe malfunction. If any of these problems in observed you should leave the sexual activity and ensure that you take necessary actions to inhibit them.

- Maintain Intimacy: Regardless of the stage of pregnancy, you should maintain intimate sessions before, during, and after pregnancy. It will make it easier to resume positions even after your partner delivers. Failure to maintain intimacy after your partner conceives may lower her self-esteem and eventually lose interest in future sex. Consequently, you would require a desperate measure to rejuvenate the mood or miss it altogether.

Pros of Sex in Pregnancy

1. Eases labor: Frequent sex sessions make it easy for the woman to give birth and recover. The contraction of muscles experienced during sex aids in strengthening the pelvic muscles. As a result, the vagina

easily opens up while resuming its previous state due to the flexibility of muscles.

2. Fewer breaks: The contractions cause muscle movements to make it easy for the vagina to hold any discharge that is associated with pregnancy. As a result, the woman can hold for long, thus requiring less time for making bathroom breaks.

3. Prevention: Engaging in sex while pregnant is beneficial for it incorporates nutrients from the sperms that aid in the growth of the unborn and the well-being of the woman. The protein found in sperms offer nutrients that help prevent pre-eclampsia.

4. Controls Blood Pressure: Sex controls your blood pressure when you are pregnant. The activity itself acts as an exercise that aids in blood circulation throughout the body, strengthening your immune system and respiration. These are essential aspects that determine your health and that of the unborn.

5. Boosts mood: It is common to experience mood swings, especially when you are pregnant. The condition worse if your

partner shows no sexual expression. For that reason, you should engage in frequent sex to maintain orgasm remain focused. Orgasm induces the circulation of blood in your pelvis, which is vital for the health of your uterus and vagina. The ripened pelvis makes it right to prepare for labor and safe delivery.

6. Improves Self-Esteem: Pregnancy comes with its effects on how you perceive yourself. The biological processes that take place during this time affect the hormonal balance hence the lowering of self-esteem. However, your partner's sexual stimulation and caressing revamp your self-confidence as you feel treasured and adored regardless of the condition.

7. Reduces Stress: The loneliness associated with pregnancy nay make a woman indulges in self-examination and worries about the unborn. The most common results are depression and stress, which could reduce through companionship and intimacy. By caring for your pregnant partner and giving

her the best sexual stimulation, you reduce her stress and refresh her mind.

8. Nurtures Your Relationship: Sex during pregnancy jakes it clear that you love your partner unconditionally. They feel endowed and appreciated knowing that they hold a precious gift in them. Finding time to connect with your partner during pregnancy boost a mutual connection which soars even after conception.

Cons

1. Premature Labor: There have been cases of premature labor in couples who engage in sex during pregnancy. The cases are high, especially if the pregnancy is on the third trimester. For this reason, you should consult your doctor before engaging in sex at this period.

2. Vaginal Bleeding: The sensitivity of the pelvis makes it prone to injury, especially if the man makes a deep penetration or hits it hard. There may be excessive bleeding putting the woman at risk of low blood

count, which is a severe condition in pregnancy.

3. Infections: Sex during pregnancy requires partners to be cautious about how they engage. Some practices could put both the mother and the unborn at risk of infections. An example would be caused by combining anal sex with vaginal sex which would bring bacteria to the pelvis and eventually affect the unborn.

4. Membrane Eruption: Deep penetration, as well as inappropriate sex positions, would lead to membrane eruption and possibly miscarriage. You should check out for signs of bleeding and pain during intercourse as warnings to these possibilities.

Best Positions for Sex During Pregnancy

- Side by side: In this position, the partners face the same direction lying by their sides with the man behind. It typically resembles the typical posture made while they sleep, leaving the bump comfortable and free. The penetration from behind offers great clit stimulation and ability to caress the woman.

- Woman on top: In this position, the woman takes full control of the depth and pace of penetration. If she sits on the flat-lying man, the bump remains suspended as she allows the man to caress her and stimulate her clitoris.
- Oral: It is a safer form off sex in pregnancy as it does not affect the formation in the pelvis. The fact that there is no penetration makes it comfortable for women who might be concerned with penetration at the time.
- Anal: It does not involve vaginal penetration and still offers sexual stimulation through be nerve endings at the anus. You should not make contact with the vaginal openings when engaging in anal sex to avoid spreading of bacterial infections.

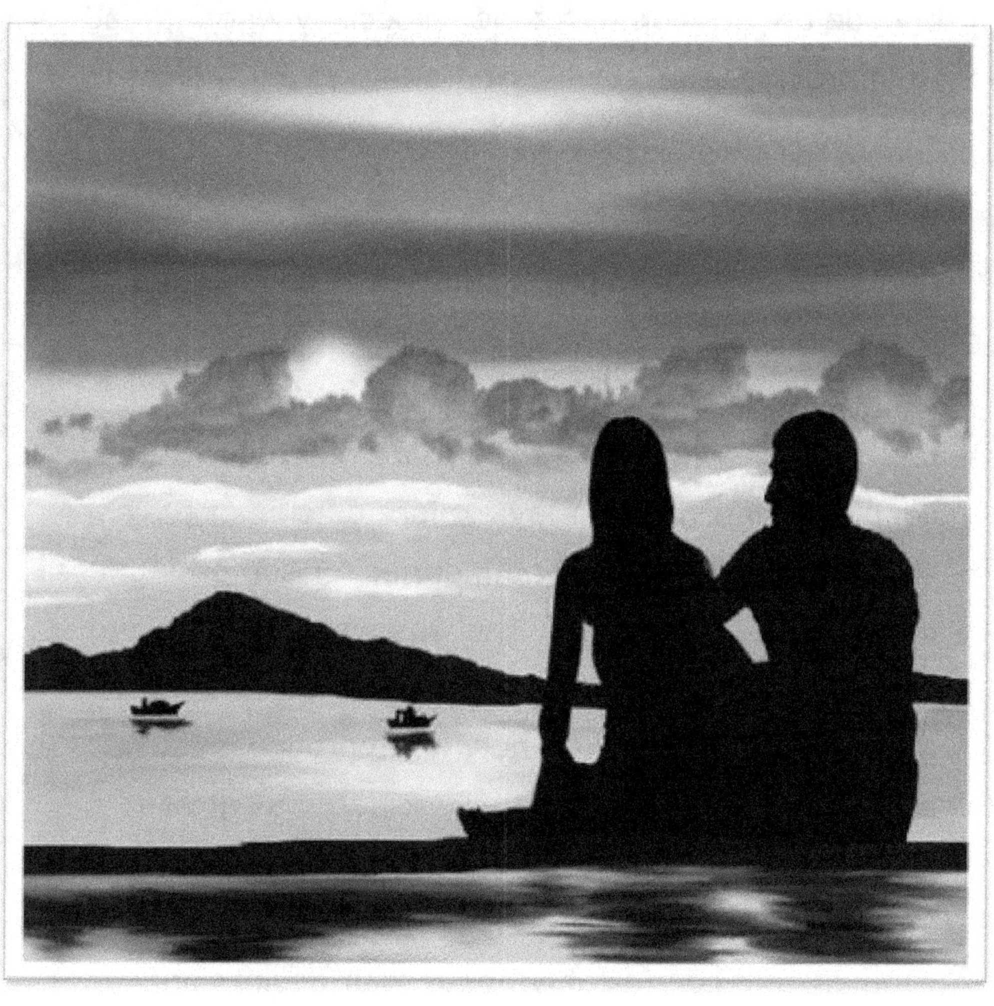

Conclusion

It is always a good idea to explore things that are outside of your comfort zone, especially when it leads to improving your sex life and bringing enjoyment to you and your partner together.

Intimacy is an important part of a healthy relationship, and people sexual needs change and evolve over time. Some couples are eager to experiment and try new techniques early in the relationship, while others are more reserved. Other couples or individuals may explore outside of their comfort zone or regular boundaries for something less conventional later in life. The way we are raised and society's view on the idea of intimacy can play a major role in influencing how we approach love, sex, and relationships. Fortunately, society has grown more accepting of a more open approach to sex and intimacy, making it easier for more people to talk candidly and comfortably about their desires and ideas.

Sometimes a small change, such as a minor adjustment in a position or a new style of oral sex, can make a tremendous boost in your sex life. Exploring something a bit different — such as a new setting, technique, or just the discussion of an idea (as subtle or wild as it may be) — can make a profound improvement in how we engage with our partner. Never underestimate the power of a simple suggestion or shared thought, even if done on a whim. If your partner shares their ideas with you, consider this as a new opportunity of fun you can explore with them or, at the very least, a good start toward communicating about your shared experiences and needs. Displaying willingness and having a partner who is on board with exploring many options is what an ideal relationship strives for. While communication and trust are the foundation of a successful relationship and intimacy, learning to accept new and exciting experiences can make a major improvement in your love life.

It is always good to still maintain the passion, excitement, fire and orgasm in a relationship; it is not always about having sex but having a sex session that it steamy, adventurous and orgasmic thrilling. So a sex session should have some spanking, naughty and very acrobatic sex styles accompanying it. You want to see your partner screaming, moaning, and being erupt in toe-curling, backing arching and orgasmic thrills then it good to learn new adventurous, crazy and deeper connection sex positions just like the ones we have in this book, there are new and thrilling sex positions that you must try out to get your partner mesmerize in the bedroom.

As earlier stated at the beginning of this book, to get you some very hot and adventurous sex positions that will aid you in your relationship I'm sure by now you would have learned a lot from all the sex positions that have been outlined for each sexual areas of your relationship. The fact is that different sex positions works for different purposes, so you should be trying the different sex position for any sexual needs you really want to achieve in your relationship. With this book we started on why you need to have sex regularly, of course sex is one of human outstanding needs that needs to be fulfilled and satisfied because it brings about emotional, mental, physical, social, intellectual and health benefits so to have your partner have memorable time with you and become obsess with your body then you should have sex with them regularly.